Achieve Your Greatness!

Achieve Your Greatness!

Squeezing the best out of what you have to offer

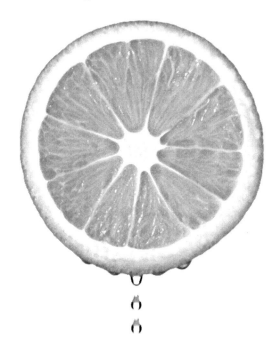

Vincenzo Aliberti, Ph.D.

Also by Dr. Vincenzo Aliberti, Ph.D.
Canadian Domestic and International Mergers and Acquisitions: A Spatial Imperfections Dimension

VAP Publishing House
Tuscany Valley Heights Northwest, Suite 101
Calgary, Alberta T3L 2E7

ISBN: 978-0-9879215-1-2
ISBN e-book: 978-0-9879215-0-5

For information regarding special discounts for bulk purchases,
please contact VAP Publishing House at valibert2000@yahoo.com

Contents

To all people,
believe in yourself
and NEVER GIVE UP!

Acknowledgements

My sincere thanks to my wife, Laureen, and my two wonderful daughters, Victoria Loren Aliberti and Isabella Julia Aliberti. I learn something new from each of you every day!

I would like to thank my father, Umberto Aliberti, my mother, Giuseppa Aliberti, my brother, Domenico Aliberti, my Zia Maria (Aunt Marie) and Zio Emilio (Uncle Emilio). Your love and support has always been there for me.

I would also like to thank the editor of this book, Kelli Taylor of KMT Solutions. Thank you for all of your suggestions Kelli.

Introduction

Achieve Your Greatness is about reaching your true potential. Many of us restrict ourselves in so many ways that we never reach our desired goals. Sure we talk a good game, but when push comes to shove, we fall short.

Take me, for example. I always looked for flaws in myself when I was younger. Maybe it was because of the way I was brought up. Perhaps it was because of the way I acted and reacted to people in my environment. Maybe it was because of the choices and non-choices I made along the way.

Because of this, I began to read a tremendous amount of personal development, personal success and self-help literature. I came to the conclusion that it was a combination of all the above. I was the way I was because of the way I was programmed, based on the environment I was in; the way I acted and reacted to people and circumstances I was in; and because of the choices and non-choices I had made along the way.

Today is a different story altogether. I have re-discovered my greatness. You see, I began focusing on a few key attributes that have made people great throughout history. These attributes were the key to re-discovering who and what I am all about. The reason why I am writing this book is not only to share these attributes with you, but to show the different faces they have. The key attributes I am speaking of are as follows:

1. Attitude

2. Courage

3. Action

4. Passion

5. Compassion

6. Perseverance

7. Leadership

8. Happiness

9. Wisdom

The list is by no means exhaustive. The aspects I have chosen to focus on in this book are based on my life, the interactions I have had with others and all of the literature I have read over the years. By the way, the last two, Happiness and Wisdom, are a result of the interactions or the combinations of the first 7.

Writing this book is my first step to reaching my true potential or greatness. To get the most out of this book, read one page, take it in, look at the perspective I am coming from, then put your spin on it. After all, each of us sees the world through different lenses. I want you to take what I write down in this book and make it yours. After reading this book, look at your life and apply what I have written in this book one minute, one hour, and one day at a time. Over time, you will notice a big change in the way you see yourself and the role you play in this world. Enjoy reading, and chart your journey to "your greatness!"

Chapter 1

ATTITUDE

Introduction

Your attitude towards yourself and others is a key determinant towards how happy or successful you are, or will be. I normally go and buy a coffee in the morning and sit down for a few minutes before I start working. I'll just sit on a bench somewhere and enjoy drinking my coffee. I see people with expensive suits come by. I see people who are living on the street pass by. I also see the gambit in between.

Whether you are rich or poor doesn't matter to me. What I find interesting are the facial expressions of all of the people who walk by. You have people living on the streets who are extremely happy, and you also find those who are thoroughly depressed. You also have those people with expensive suits who are happy, but then again you find those who are absolutely miserable. When everything is said and done, one major reason why someone is happy is because of his/her attitude, or outlook on life.

After you read the section on attitude, take a good look in the mirror and see whether you need to modify your attitude to a certain extent, or if your outlook is where it should be. Not to ruin the ending, but we all need to gauge and recalibrate our attitude toward life once in a while, otherwise we never grow.

Attitudes towards obstacles!

*"If you don't like something, change it.
If you can't change it, change your attitude."*

~ *Maya Angelou*

Marguerite Ann Johnson, better known as Maya Angelou, is an American author and poet. She is best known for her six autobiographical volumes that focus on her childhood and early adult experiences.

Maya, as well as many African-Americans, were regarded as second-class citizens during the civil rights movement that took place in the 1960s. Many times she fought an uphill battle. She knew life was a challenge.

Like Maya, we also know life is not a bed of roses. We, too, have obstacles each and every day. What distinguishes one person from another is their attitude towards that obstacle. As Maya states, "If you don't like something, change it. If you can't change it, change your attitude." For many, they never change their attitude until it is too late. Are you one of them?

Attitude and breaking free!

"So often time it happens, we all live our life in chains, and we never even know we have the key."

~The Eagles

The Eagles are an American rock band that was formed in Los Angeles, California in 1971. For some, they are considered one of the greatest bands of all time. The original members of the band were Glenn Frey, Don Henley, Bernie Leadon and Randy Meisner.

How profound is their quote? Each one of us never really takes a good look at how good we have it until it is too late. We pout and complain by saying "I wish I had this," or "I wish I had that." The fact of the matter is, we have to do the best with what we have.

Some people look at a glass and say the glass is half empty, while others say it is half full. We really need to take the time to check the way we see our life. We need to look at the positive aspects of life. To do that, we need to change our attitude toward life. Should we go through life and live in chains, or break free from the chains that we create ourselves? I know what I want; how about you?

Attitude and assumptions!

"Begin challenging your own assumptions. Your assumptions are your windows on the world. Scrub them off every once in a while, or the light won't come in."

~ Alan Alda

Alphonso Joseph D'Abruzzo, better known as Alan Alda, is an American actor, director, screenwriter, and author. He is best known for his role as Hawkeye Pierce in the TV series M*A*S*H.

Just glance up and re-read Alan Alda's quote once again. For me, the word WOW comes to mind. Let's face it, from the time we are born until the time we reach adulthood, we are taught what is right, what is wrong, what to do, and what not to do. Our worldly beliefs are founded on the assumptions of others. In essence, we see the world we live in through a certain pair of lenses.

Once in a while, we need to re-visit what we have been taught. We need to change our 'attitude' towards how we view things. I challenge myself at least one time a day to re-visit the way I view things. I try to change my 'attitude' towards the way I see the world. I scrub my lenses once a day. My question is, do you?

Meaning lies in attitude!

"The meaning of things lies not in the things themselves, but in our attitude towards them."

~ Antoine de Saint-Exupery

Antoine de Saint-Exupéry was a prominent French writer, poet and pioneering aviator. He is best remembered for his novella "The Little Prince," and for his lyrical aviation writings, "Night Flight" and "Wind, Sand and Starts."

Saint-Exupéry had attitude in spades. He was a great writer, but many people don't know that he was a commercial pilot for France during WW II. He had an air that he could accomplish anything he set his mind to. He realized that in order to get the most out of life, he had to attach attitude to the meaning of things he valued.

To get the most out of life we need to imbed that attitude into our moral fibre. We can reach new heights by empowering ourselves with the way we add meaning to every aspect of our life. Now, I am not saying we will accomplish everything we set out to accomplish, but we will probably come pretty close.

What the mind can conceive and believe, it can achieve!

"What the mind of man can conceive and believe, it can achieve."

~ Napolean Hill

Napoleon Hill was one of the greatest writers on "success literature." His most famous work, *Think and Grow Rich*, sold over 20 million copies by 1970, the time of his death. In *Think and Grow Rich*, Hill provided a formula on how an average person can achieve new heights. This formula is still applied by many people today. Napoleon was truly ahead of his time.

I can definitely relate to Napoleon's quote. Many times throughout my life I have doubted myself. I simply felt I was not able to accomplish certain things. I was not in the right frame of mind. My "attitude" was all wrong! I conceived what I wanted to do, *but I did not believe it*, and therefore I did not achieve it.

However, almost every time I really believed in whatever I conceived, I achieved. What did I do that was different? I changed my "attitude." Remember, we control our destiny. Make your mind work for you. Conceive high goals and dreams for yourself. Believe that you will reach your goals and attain your dreams. Achieve your goals and dreams one small step at a time! What Napoleon says in his quote has worked for millions of people. Change your attitude and make it work for you!

Attitude and prison bars!

"Two men look out the same prison bars;
one sees mud and the other stars."

~ *Frederick Langbridge*

Frederick Langbridge was born in Birmingham, England. He became a Reverend in 1877. Reverend Langbridge was also a writer, poet (*The Scales of Heaven*) and playwright (*The Only Way*).

Every time I go to a family function I bump across some family members who are really happy just to be there. Other family members may have a problem here and there and they voice it out, but they are still generally happy. Then there are those who constantly complain about everything. They think that nothing is going right for them. I am sure you have people in your family, or even friends or acquaintances like that.

The constant complainers about life create their own prison through their negative attitude. To top it all off, they want to pass it on to you. If people want to create and live in their own prisons they are more than welcome. After all, it is their choice. When people with negative attitudes look at prison bars they see mud. When I look at prison bars I see stars. What do you see?

Attitude and altitude!

"It is your attitude, not your aptitude that determines your altitude."

~ Zig Ziglar

Zig Ziglar was born in Coffee County, Alabama. He is an American author, salesman, and motivational speaker. In 1968 he became a vice president and training director of an automotive organization. He later turned to professional speaking full-time.

When you look at yourself you can probably find one thing you are really good at. Some of us are good athletes, painters, police officers, physicists, good communicators, writers, or plumbers. My point is that we have something special in each and every one of us, whatever that something is. Some of us may be good at what we do, others are phenomenal at what they do. What distinguishes the two individuals? In one word, 'attitude.'

If you are good at your craft, but your attitude towards it is less than stellar, then you will probably not reach the heights you were destined to reach. On the other hand, if your attitude is stellar, then the likelihood of your reaching your heights increases significantly. After all, it's like Zig says, "It is your attitude, not your aptitude that determines your altitude!"

Change your attitude;
let things go!

"Holding on to anger is like grasping a hot coal with the intent of throwing it at someone else; you are the one who gets burned."

~ Buddha

Siddhartha Gautama (Buddha) was said to have been born in the small state of Kapilavastu, which is now Nepal. He was a spiritual teacher who traveled and taught throughout India, and on whose teachings Buddhism was founded. He was often referred to as the Supreme Buddha. "Buddha" means "awakened one" or "enlightened one."

Ever wonder why people get irritated? Ever wonder why some people let the smallest things get to them? Ever wonder why people walk around with a chip on their shoulder? Well I don't have to wonder, because I was one of those people. I was always so angry about something. I made my problems bigger than they were. Since then, I have come a long way!

I have three really good friends, let's call them Diano, Konrad and Ray. These guys are cool as cucumbers. Whatever happens to them, they let it go. They know they cannot change the past. They deal with things accordingly. To reference Buddha's quote, they don't hold onto anger like hot coal, so they don't get burned. What about you?

Attitude and the real you!

"Seek out that particular mental attribute which makes you feel most deeply and vitally alive, along with which comes the inner voice which says, "This is the real me," and when you have found that attitude, follow it."

~ James Truslow Adams

James Truslow Adams was an American writer and historian. Adams received his bachelor's degree from the Polytechnic Institute of Brooklyn, and master's degree from Yale University. He began working as an investment banker. Once he saved enough money he decided to switch his career and follow his passion, writing.

Adams' quote is quite inspiring. It's inspiring because it talks about how your attitude can make you come ALIVE! How your attitude brings out the real you! Hey, how many times have you truly not been yourself at a social function, business meeting, or with your friends and family members? I believe most of us have had this experience. It all goes back to your attitude. Our attitude towards a given situation greatly impacts the way we see ourselves in the situation we are in. Your inner voice knows it, and makes sure you are not yourself in that situation.

To truly share yourself with others, you first need to feel comfortable in your own shoes. You need to change your attitude towards things. Once you do that, you will truly be alive with yourself and the rest of the world!

Attitude and successful outcomes!

"It is our attitude at the beginning of a difficult task which, more than anything else, will affect its successful outcome."

-*William James*

William James was born in New York City. He was a pioneering psychologist and philosopher who was trained as a physician. He wrote influential books on variety of subjects, some of which include: educational psychology, psychology of religious experience and mysticism, and the philosophy of pragmatism.

Do me a favour, carefully read his quote once again. For me, three words automatically come to mind: 'attitude,' 'beginning,' and 'outcome.' Let's face it, whether you are changing a baby's diapers or working on a major home renovation project, the principle is still the same. With a positive 'attitude' in the 'beginning,' as you execute what you need to do, you will be more fulfilled with the 'outcome.' Conversely, if you have a poor attitude in the 'beginning,' and you execute what you need to do, you will be less fulfilled with the 'outcome.'

Look at starting off on the right foot. A positive attitude at the beginning will set the tone of anything to come, and will increase the likelihood of success in whatever you do. Positive attitude breeds positive energy. Negative attitude breeds negative energy. I suggest we focus on the positive here. What do you think?

Chapter Summary

ATTITUDE

1. If you don't like something, change it. If you can't change it, change your attitude.

2. Break free from your self-imposed prison.

3. Scrub your assumptions once in a while.

4. Meaning is not in the things themselves, but in our attitude towards them.

5. What the mind can conceive and believe, it can achieve!

6. Make sure you see stars when you look at prison bars.

7. Your attitude determines your altitude!

8. Let the past be the past. Start living for today.

9. Let the real you shine through. Be and act vitally alive.

10. Focus on the positive, it will serve you better in whatever you want to accomplish.

Personal Notes on "Attitude"

1. _____

   _____

   _____

   _____

2. _____

   _____

   _____

   _____

3. _____

   _____

   _____

   _____

4. _____

   _____

   _____

   _____

   _____

5. _____

   _____

   _____

   _____

Chapter 2

COURAGE

Introduction

You know the saying, 'Leaders are made, not born.' That is how I feel about the word courage. Courage is something some people have more of than others, but those who don't have as much can gain it over time. Those individuals simply have to place themselves in uncomfortable situations, and get used to being uncomfortable.

I strongly believe if you have a realistic view of the world around you, and calibrate your attitude to that realism, then courage is simply another step, or extension, that needs to be taken in your journey through life. What distinguishes you from someone else is that extra step.

Courage and not speaking!

*"Courage is what it takes to stand up and
speak; courage is also what it takes to sit
down and listen."*

~ *Winston Churchill*

Sir Winston Leonard Spencer-Churchill was a British politician and statesman. He is known for his leadership of the United Kingdom during the Second World War. He is widely regarded as one of the greatest wartime leaders of the century and served as Prime Minister twice. He was an avid writer and received the Nobel Prize in Literature.

As a politician, Churchill knew when to open his mouth and say something, and when not to open his mouth at all. Over time, I'm sure he fine-tuned what to say when. Now, there are people who talk all of the time. There are those who refuse to talk at all. There are some who are somewhere in between. There are merits to all three, depending on the circumstances. However, here I am going to focus on those people who talk a lot, all the time.

It takes a great deal of courage to state your opinions. Why do I say that? Well, I have a fear of speaking in public, but I have improved over the years. So, I have a great deal of respect for people who voice their opinions. It's liberating to express your facts and opinion to others. It's great to say what is on your mind in a one-on-one, or group environment. However, when you go over the top, it's just simply annoying. Like Winston Churchill states, "Courage is what it takes to stand up and speak; courage is also what it takes to sit down and listen." I have learned a tremendous amount more when I 'truly listened' than when I spoke. How about you?

Courage and fear!

"Courage is resistance to fear, mastery of fear, not absence of fear."

~ Mark Twain

Samuel Langhorne Clemens, better known as Mark Twain, was an American author. He is most noted for his novels, The Adventures of Tom Sawyer, and its sequel, Adventures of Huckleberry Finn. The latter is often called "the Great American Novel." He earned a tremendous amount of praise for his wit and satire from both critics and peers.

If any of you say to me you have never been scared in your lives, I would call you a liar. Let's face it, we are all human. We are not perfect. Many boys, girls, men and women are fearful of public speaking. I fall into that category. Bottom line, everyone has their own fears. Some of us choose to deal with them, while others do not.

I challenge you to wake up every morning and confront one of your fears, whatever it may be. By consistently confronting what you did not want to confront, over time that fear will become less of a fear, or may disappear entirely. I have joined Toastmasters, a group that helps people break out of the fear they have with public speaking. Why not confront your fear, and master it, for that matter, so you can truly live your life to the fullest?

Courage and morality!

"There are no easy answers, but there are simple answers. We must have the courage to do what we know is morally right."

~ Ronald Reagan

Ronald Wilson Reagan was born in Tampico, Illinois. Reagan was the 40th President of the United States (served two terms), the 33rd Governor of California and, prior to that, a radio, film and television actor.

As we are growing up, we are taught what is morally right from parents, or teachers, or policemen, or our spiritual leaders. However, as we are growing and continue to grow, we are also bombarded with information from friends, family, work colleagues, newspapers, television, the Internet, you name it. It's a challenge for anyone to organize and process all of that information.

When you couple the way you were brought up with the information we are inundated with on a daily basis, sometimes it's difficult to distinguish what is morally right or wrong. I believe in the goodness of people around the world. However, no matter how good people are, even their moral compass can be off a couple of degrees here and there. Make sure to check your moral compass once in a while. You may have to tweak it to determine where you are, or where you want to be.

Courage, purpose and direction!

"Efforts and courage are not enough without purpose and direction."

~ *John F. Kennedy*

John "Jack" Fitzgerald, often referred to by his initials JFK, was the 35th President of the United States, serving from 1961 until his assassination in 1963. Kennedy was the only Catholic president, and the only president to have won a Pulitzer Prize. Today, Kennedy continues to rank highly in public opinion ratings of former U.S. presidents.

When I was a kid I put in tons of effort trying to improve my soccer skills, and given that I played goalie, I knew I had tons of courage as well. I used to get up every morning and do 500 push-ups, 500 sit-ups, and run for a few miles. Mind you, I was 16 at the time. I later went on to get a soccer scholarship to Oakland University, and I even played semi-professional soccer in Canada.

I put in the effort, and I had the courage to face any obstacle in front of me. I also had purpose and direction. I fell short of my goal because I wanted to play professional soccer in Europe, but that is okay. I did the best I could with what I had at the time. Regardless of your chosen field, you can be the best you can be if you put in the effort, are courageous, and have purpose and direction! Why not give yourself that chance?

Meeting things head on!

"You have to accept whatever comes, and the only important thing is that you meet it with courage and with the best that you have to give."

~ Eleanor Roosevelt

Anna Eleanor Roosevelt was the First Lady of the United States from 1933 to 1945. Roosevelt was an author, speaker, politician, and civil rights activist. Her work enhanced the status of working women around the globe.

I have learned over the years that by shying away from things, I simply dug a bigger hole for myself. In family gatherings I would not speak. At work, in team meetings, I would rarely say anything. In short, I would not share my thoughts because it was easier for me to be standoffish, and stay in the background.

One day I said to myself, enough is enough. I said to myself I was going to have the courage to say what I needed to say in a polite and professional manner. Once I met my fear head-on, it became a habit over time, and I haven't looked back. No matter what I am confronted with nowadays, I know I can conquer it if I meet it head on. I am sure you can do the same. Meet things head on!

...and justification!

...the courage will always
...philosophy to justify it."

~ *Albert Camus*

Albert Camus was a French author, journalist, and key philosopher of the 20th century. He was the first African-born writer to receive the Nobel Prize in Literature. His literary work brought to life the problems of the human conscience as seen through his eyes.

How many times have you found yourself saying, 'I am going to start weight watchers next year because I have so many things in my life right now?' How about, 'I'll stop drinking or smoking in a few weeks?' How many different New Year's resolutions have you made, and never 'fully' followed through on? Yeah, you may have started, but never completed what you set out to do. Oh yeah, and we always have an excuse for why we stopped.

If you keep on doing what you have always done, you will get the same results you have always received. When you start something, have the courage to carry it through. Just start it today. It's easy to make excuses and think you're getting away with something. Reach the goals and dreams you want! Stop making excuses!

Courage and dreams!

"It takes a lot of courage to show your dreams to someone else."

~ Erma Bombeck

Erma Louise Bombeck was an American author and newspaper columnist. From 1965 to 1996, Bombeck wrote over 4,000 newspaper columns about the ordinary life of a Midwestern suburban housewife. Bombeck also published 15 books, most of which became best-sellers.

People have always told me to keep things close to your vest. Well, to a certain degree they are right. Let's face it, there are people who simply do not want you to succeed. Why, you say? Well, maybe they are afraid you won't be friends with them anymore. Perhaps they don't have the confidence in themselves to see things through, and they don't want you to follow through either. There are tons of reasons why people don't want you to succeed. Mind you, there are also many reasons people do want you to succeed.

It's taking me a while to realize it's alright for me to show my dreams to someone else. Whether they choose to support me or not, that's okay. I know who my true friends are, and you know yours. Have the courage to share your dreams with others! Have the courage to realize your dreams, with or without others!

Courage and truth, morality and integrity!

"Have the courage to say no. Have the courage to face the truth. Do the right thing because it is right. These are the magic keys to living your life with integrity."

~ W. Clement Stone

William Clement Stone was a businessman, philanthropist and New Thought self-help book author. He ended up turning $100 into millions by applying the principles from Napoleon Hills' book, *Think and Grow Rich*. His motto was "Whatever the mind can conceive and believe, the mind can achieve with a positive mental attitude."

No matter who you are in this world, you live in a cage. What do I mean by that? Well, all of us think what we experience is really the way the world is, given the lenses we see the world through. As a result, we have our own definition of truth, morality and integrity.

Over time, some people challenge their definition of truth, morality and integrity, while others do not. Some of us grow faster than others. Some of us simply don't want to grow at all. Some of us fall somewhere in between. Find the truths about your truths, your moral values and your true integrity. You may be surprised with what you will find out about yourself, I know I did.

Courage and causes!

"Many a man will have the courage to die gallantly, but will not have the courage to say, or even to think, that the cause for which he is asked to die is an unworthy one."

~ Bertrand Russell

Bertrand Arthur William Russell was born in Monmouthshire, into one of the most prominent aristocratic families in Britain. He was a British philosopher, logician, mathematician, historian, and social critic. In 1950, Russell was awarded the Nobel Prize in Literature.

I have the greatest admiration for people who have the courage, direction and purpose to reach and realize their goals and dreams. Whether you are a parent, entrepreneur, chief executive officer, or an officer in a non-profit organization, all of you have specific goals in mind. For the parent, it may be to raise healthy kids who contribute to society. For the entrepreneur, it may be to patent his/her innovation and start a business. For the chief executive officer, it may be to improve shareholder returns. For the officer working in a non-profit organization, it may be to help feed and clothe the poor.

It takes a great deal of courage to say to yourself 'this is what I want and I am going to go for it.' Have the courage to take that first step, because if you don't, you'll have no idea what you will be missing.

Courage and opposites!

"This soul, or life within us, by no means agrees with the life outside us. If one has the courage to ask her what she thinks, she is always saying the very opposite to what other people say."

~ *Virginia Woolf*

Adeline Virginia Woolf was an English author, essayist, publisher, and writer of short stories. She is considered one of the most prominent literary geniuses of the twentieth century. Some of her most famous works include the novels *Mrs. Dalloway, To the Lighthouse*, and *Orlando*.

Many times in our lives we conform. When you are in a group with your friends, rather than stir the pot, you go along with what everyone else wants. When you are at a meeting at work, you don't want to stir the pot because you don't want to upset your manager. There are many examples to include here.

Hey, there is a time and a place to say certain things. When that time and place comes, have the courage to express your facts and/or opinions. Stop holding yourself back! Have the courage to express yourself and set yourself free!

Chapter Summary

COURAGE

1. You can learn a great deal by just listening.

2. Master your fear, or your fear will master you.

3. Do what is morally right.

4. Obtain your dreams through your courage, purpose and direction.

5. Don't shy away from your obstacles, confront them.

6. Just do it. Don't justify your lack of courage.

7. Show people your dreams, but don't get deterred.

8. Find the truths about your truths, morality and integrity.

9. Fight for what your worthy beliefs!

10. Don't live a lie. Let your interior and exterior match!

Personal Notes on "Courage"

1. _____
   _____
   _____
   _____

2. _____
   _____
   _____
   _____

3. _____
   _____
   _____
   _____

4. _____

_____

_____

_____

_____

5. _____

_____

_____

_____

Chapter 3

ACTION

Introduction

If you take two runners, one who starts running once the starting gun sounds, and one who remains still on the starting line once the gun sounds, the odds are that the guy who is running towards the finish line is going to win. Okay, I am exaggerating here, but you get my point. With action, you get results. With inaction, although it is an action in itself, you get limited results.

It's been proven throughout history that inventors have failed hundreds, even thousands of times before they get their invention right. However, these inventors acted and eventually got to their desired goal. Without action you will simply be where you are right now, with maybe a slight change. Put your thoughts into action; it will serve you well in the long run.

Thinking and action!

"Take time to deliberate; but when the time for action arrives, stop thinking and go in."

~ *Napoleon Bonaparte*

Napoleon Bonaparte was born in Corsica. Educated at military school, he was rapidly promoted and in 1796, was made commander of the French army in Italy. He is considered one of the greatest military leaders in history. As the emperor of France, he conquered much of Europe.

I remember when I was doing my doctorate. I just loved the process of trying to find alternative solutions to a given problem. In all honesty, I loved the process of finding alternatives so much that it ended up taking so much longer to reach a solution. Now, just imagine a painter who wants to create a painting. The painter knows exactly what he/she wants to paint, but has a difficult time determining the colors the painting should be comprised of. What is wrong with this picture? Well, the painter doesn't get to finish his/her painting until a much later date.

There is nothing wrong with thinking things through. There is nothing wrong with being exacting in your approach. However, you don't want to get analysis-paralysis. In other words, don't get stuck in what you are doing and never take action! Think about what needs to be done and take action!

Action and urgency!

"I have been impressed with the urgency of doing. Knowing is not enough; we must apply. Being willing is not enough; we must do."

~ Leonardo da Vinci

Leonardo di ser Piero da Vinci was an Italian Renaissance polymath: painter, sculptor, architect, musician, scientist, mathematician, engineer, inventor, anatomist, geologist, cartographer, botanist and writer. During his time, he was a true Renaissance man.

I, like you, have known people who run around, and around, and around, and accomplish practically nothing. I have also worked with people who run around and achieve practically everything they want to accomplish. It's great that people know what needs to be done. It's great they take action to do what needs to be done. It's great they do it with urgency.

Before you take action, take a deep breath. Think about what you are going to do, why you are going to do it, and how you are going to do it. Next, and this is just as important, know when you are going to action it. There is no point running all over the place to accomplish what needs to be done, if you don't know when you are going to act. More importantly, if you know when you are going to act, do so with urgency. That way, you have immediately acted once you have made a decision to act, and there is no looking back. The last thing you want is to say you are going to do something, and then do nothing. It is that split second of urgency after you have made the decision to act that will take you from inaction to action. So, act with urgency!

Knowing yourself through action!

"To know oneself is to study oneself in action with another person."

~ Bruce Lee

Bruce Lee was born in San Francisco, United States. He was a martial arts instructor, philosopher, actor, film director, film producer, screenwriter, and founder of the Jeet Kune Do martial arts movement. Bruce was considered a cultural icon during his time.

Do you know people who say, "I am so awesome at my job, I am going to get a promotion soon?" Do you know people who say, "You know, I am going to lose 50 pounds by this time next year?" These are the people who say they are going to do this, and then they are going to do that, and have a hard time accomplishing anything. I know a few of these people. I am sure you know a few as well.

One thing I believe is that "talk is cheap." Each and every one of us can talk trash if we want to. My point here is, if you say you are going to do something, do it! If you say you are going to do something, take action! If you don't take action, whatever you want to do is simply going to be a pipe dream. If you conceive, believe, and act, you will achieve!

Action and intelligence!

"Action is the real measure of intelligence."

~ Napoleon Hill

Napoleon Hill was one of the greatest writers on "success literature." His most famous work, *Think and Grow Rich*, sold over 20 million copies by 1970, the time of his death. In *Think and Grow Rich*, Hill provided a formula about how an average person can achieve new heights. This formula is still applied by many people today.

Let's talk about two groups of people I have known in my life. In the first group, you have those who have a tremendous amount of intelligence and potential, but simply had a challenging time realizing their goals. In the second group, you have people who are intelligent, with far less pure potential than the first group, but who seemed to realize their goals more often than not. So, what distinguishes the people in these two groups? Those in the first group thought too much and took steps at a snail's pace to try to realize their dreams. Those in the second group thought about things for just the right amount of time, were fully committed, and acted at a much faster pace.

To put my own personal spin on it, one thing about me is I am an ideas guy and a strategist. When I was younger, it would take a while for me to act. Yeah, I would think intelligently about things, but used to take those very, very, very small steps as I was going forward. Today I am a different man, I think intelligently, and then act wholeheartedly! More often than not I achieve the desired results. Use your intelligence wisely, think, then act! Don't miss your window of opportunity!

Action and reaction!

*"The possibilities are numerous once we
decide to act and not react."*

~ *George Bernard Shaw*

George Bernard Shaw was an Irish playwright and a co-founder of the London School of Economics in the United Kingdom. His major claim to fame was his innate ability to write incredible dramas. He wrote over 60 during his lifetime. Shaw works were about education, marriage, religion, government, health care, and class privilege.

I was born in Taormina, Sicily in Italy. I know there is a stereotype out there that all Italians are passionate and react to everything. Well, let me set the record straight. Maybe some Italians are passionate and react to everything, but there are also those who are not as passionate and react to nothing. I am very passionate, and 'act' accordingly. Notice that I didn't say 'react,' but 'act' accordingly. Yes, sometimes I react, but I try to minimize that, because in the grand scheme of things it does not serve me well.

By taking in information throughout our day, organizing it, and 'acting' on it accordingly, one can lead a more tranquil life. Conversely, by taking in information throughout our day, organizing it, and 'reacting,' one can lead a more stressful life. These are two possibilities regarding how one can live their life based on what I have just written. As I have stated a few times in this book, the choice is ultimately yours.

Action and ignorance!

*"There is nothing more frightful than
ignorance in action."*

~ *Johann Wolfgang von Goethe*

Johann Wolfgang von Goethe was a German writer, pictorial artist, biologist, theoretical physicist, and polymath. His works span the fields of poetry, drama, prose, philosophy, and science. He is considered the supreme genius of modern German literature.

Goethe's quote really puts things in perspective, if perspective is what you are looking for. Many times in our lives we go about our day thinking we know exactly what we are getting into. Some examples of that are: investing in financial instruments we think are going to make us some money, or stereotyping people who are different from us because of something we have seen on television or the Internet. What are we doing when this occurs? Many times, we think we are acting on what we perceive to be the truth. What is really happening is we are acting and saying things based on limited information. To top it all off, some of the time, the information we are getting is from a non-reputable, or should I say, less reputable source.

Making sure you have the most pertinent and relevant information before you act is extremely important, but check the true accuracy of it as well. Accuracy means how close we are to the actual truth. Let's not be ignorant before we act; let's get the facts straight and act without being ignorant!

Action and possibilities!

"Act as if it were impossible to fail"

~ Dorothea Brande

Dorothea Brande was born in Chicago, Illinois and attended the University of Chicago, the Lewis Institute (modern day Illinois Institute of Technology), and the University of Michigan. She was a well-respected writer and editor in New York.

When I was younger I worked on an automotive assembly line for a few years. I gained invaluable life experience working "the line." I wanted something more, so I decided to get my doctorate and started working for a firm based out of Ann Arbor, Michigan. All my family and friends said I should just settle.

For some people, settling is fine. For others, settling simply does not cut it. I fall in the second category. I always strive to push myself to the next level. I live in the now, but I believe in possibilities. I believe you need to 'act' at the right time, in order to make your possibilities a reality. If you believe nothing is possible, then nothing is possible! If you believe nothing is impossible, then everything is possible!

Action, risk and truth!

"Risk! Risk anything! Care no more for the opinions of others, for those voices. Do the hardest thing on earth for you. Act for yourself. Face the truth."

~ *Katherine Mansfield*

Kathleen Mansfield Beauchamp Murry was a prominent modernist writer who was born and brought up in colonial New Zealand. She wrote under her pen name, Katherine Mansfield. Some of her famous works include; *The Garden Party, The Daughters of the Late Colonel,* and *The Fly.*

Some of the hardest choices we face occur when we are young. Our parents, teachers, or anyone we look up to want us to do one thing, but we want to do something else. When you are young, I can see how it can be difficult to not care about the opinions of others. You think highly of those people and respect their opinions. However, there is a certain age, and it varies for everyone, when we have to make decisions for ourselves. We have to create own path.

When you start creating "your own path," it is alright to get opinions from others. It is fine to ask for guidance to a certain extent. It's alright to be afraid of what may happen based on the decisions you are about to make. It's not alright for you to follow a path because someone else wants you to do so. I know this because that is exactly what I did. Luckily for me, I was able to turn things around quickly enough and proceed on the path I wanted to pursue. Don't let what happened to me happen to you. Take action and follow your path. Take calculated risks and follow your truth!

Action and results!

*"You may never know what results come
of your action, but if you do nothing there
will be no result"*

~ Mahatma Gandhi

Mohandas Karamchand Gandhi was the political and ideological leader of India during the Indian independence movement. His philosophy was founded on "total non-violence." HHGandhi led India to independence and inspired movements for human freedom across the world.

I have searched the Internet and read a great deal about Ghandi. I watched the Gandhi the movie, but I am sure it does not do him justice. That he led India to independence with a philosophy that was founded on total non-violence is absolutely incredible, if you think about it. Although India reached independence through the philosophy of non-violence, the citizens of India still 'acted' in a non-violent manner to reach their desired goals of independence and freedom.

Similar to Gandhi and the people of India, we need to act to get results. If you have a goal or a dream you want to obtain, staring at the sky won't help. Thinking about it and not doing anything about it won't help. What you and I need to do is to act on what we are thinking about, in order for us to potentially achieve our desired result. Like Ghandi states, "You may never know what results come of your action, but if you do nothing, there will be no result." Take action; you'll be grateful later that you did.

Action and success!

*"Success seems to be connected with action.
Successful people keep moving. They make
mistakes, but they don't quit."*

~ Conrad Hilton

Conrad Nicholson Hilton was born in San Antonio, New Mexico. He was an American businessman and investor. Hilton was best known for being the founder of the Hilton Hotels chain, and for his philanthropic efforts.

As I have said numerous times in this book, each of us has had our ups and downs. What distinguishes successful people from less successful people is their ability to act. Before I go further, I want you to imagine yourself as a true success as defined by you, not others. Keep that image in your mind, and think of the following words: action, moving, and quitting.

I am going to use these three words to define success. Let's face it, if you have a goal you want to reach you have to create a plan to get there. In order to obtain your desired goal you have to 'act' with purpose. Although you may encounter bumps along the way, as long as you keep on 'moving' toward your goal, you are doing well. Sometimes it takes a little longer, but the key is that you are 'moving' towards it. Next, never, ever, 'quit!' Have you ever heard of a 100 metres dash sprinter running 99 metres and winning the race? The resounding answer is NO. So, imagine you are that sprinter. The action is that you are sprinting, keep on moving toward the finish line, and don't quit before you get to the finish line. That's success in a nutshell. All you have to do is apply what I have said to the different aspects of your life.

Summary

ACTION

1. Think before acting, but when the time comes, act!

2. Get the ball rolling; apply what you know.

3. Study yourself in action with someone else.

4. Action is the real measure of intelligence.

5. The possibilities are numerous once we decide to act.

6. There is nothing more frightful than ignorance in action.

7. Act as if you are going to succeed.

8. Act by taking calculated risk to find *your* truth and realize *your* dreams.

9. Coordinate your actions to achieve your desired results.

10. Successful people keep moving.

Personal Notes on "Action"

1. _____

   _____

   _____

   _____

2. _____

   _____

   _____

   _____

3. _____

   _____

   _____

   _____

4. _____

_____

_____

_____

_____

5. _____

_____

_____

_____

Chapter 4

PASSION

Introduction

Whenever I'm passionate about something, I feel nothing can stop me. I'm sure you feel exactly the same about the things you are passionate about. As you read this, pick one thing you are passionate about. When you do that "one thing," doesn't it make you happy? Of course it does!

In life, there are things we need to do, and then there are things we are passionate about doing. Ideally we would all like to just do what we are passionate about, but as many of you know, that may be a challenge, given our current circumstances.

For some, it seems as though every moment of every waking day they are living their dream. For most of us, that is not the case. The key is to move the gauge slightly, from the things you need to do, to the things we are passionate about, as much as you can every day. By having the attitude and courage to find your passion, only happiness can follow for you.

Passion and commitment!

"Anyone can dabble, but once you've made that commitment, your blood has that particular thing in it, and it's very hard for people to stop you."

~ Bill Cosby

William Henry "Bill" Cosby Jr. is an American comedian, actor, author, television producer, educator, musician and activist. Following a brilliant stand-up comedy career, he starred in I Spy, The Cosby Show, and produced A Different World. Cosby also has a Doctorate of Education from the University of Massachusetts.

I consider myself to be quite fortunate in the sense that when I make I commitment, that's it. Whether it's trying out for a soccer team, working for a given company, my educational pursuits, or my life with my wife and kids, I can honestly say I have passion and commitment. Just like I stated previously, I feel very blessed in this regard.

When you are passionate about something so much it becomes a part of you, and you are committed to it, that's one of the best feelings in the world. With passion and commitment it's almost impossible for anyone to stop you from reaching your goals!

Passion and energy!

*"Without passion you don't have energy,
without energy you have nothing."*

~ *Donald Trump*

Donald John Trump, Sr. is a successful business magnate, television personality and author. He is the currently the chairman and president of The Trump Organization, and the founder of Trump Entertainment Resorts. Trump's outspoken personality can be seen on NBC's reality show The Apprentice.

When you find something you are passionate about, you want to do it all the time. When I first started writing this book I said to myself I would write one good page every two days for a year. I followed this plan to a tee because I was not in any rush to publish my book. Then, because I got into it so much, I had the energy to write five pages per day. I got up at 5:00 in the morning and worked for two hours, and I put in an hour after work. I had the passion and the resulting energy for it!

Find something you are really passionate about. Find something you are committed to. You will be surprised at how much energy you will have to carry through with your plan. Passion and energy make a fabulous combo; make them work for you!

Passion and reason!

*"If passion drives you,
let reason hold the reins."*

~ Benjamin Franklin

Dr. Benjamin Franklin was one of the Founding Fathers of the United States. A noted polymath, Franklin was a leading author, civic activist, diplomat, inventor, musician, politician, satirist, scientist, and statesman.

Having passion in whatever you do is fantastic. Passion is the fuel that makes your goals attainable. Passion drives people to succeed. Passion can also be destructive if not channelled accordingly. As Benjamin Franklin states, "If passion drives you, let reason hold the reins."

Just imagine you are driving a Ferrari around a race track. Now, let's say you are really putting your foot on the gas and you are about to go around one of the corners. If you are driven by passion, and not in control, when you go around that corner you will hit the wall. Whereas, if you are driving that Ferrari and you know you are almost at the corner, you slow down so you can make it without any problems. Life is the same way; have that passion and drive, use reason to control yourself, so you don't end up out of control.

Passion and Playing Small!

"There is no passion to be found playing small - in settling for a life that is less than the one you are capable of living."

~ *Nelson Mandela*

Nelson Rolihlahla Mandela served as President of South Africa from 1994 to 1999, and was the first South African president to be elected in a fully representative democratic election. As president, he frequently introduced policies aimed at combating poverty and inequality. In 1993, Mandela received the Nobel Peace Prize.

I have met some confident people in my life. I have also met people in my life who have little to no confidence. What I have noticed is that even if a confident person does not know something very well, because of his/her confidence, it will seem as though they have everything figured out. On the flip side of the coin are those individuals who know much more than the confident person, but because they are not confident in themselves, they seem as though they haven't figured out what they were supposed to figure out.

Going forward, this is what I would like you to do. First, believe in yourself and what you are capable of. Next, be passionate about what you plan to do. Last, stop playing small! You know, only you can instil or remove confidence from yourself; nobody else can. Start playing big and live up to your potential!

Passion and youth!

"Passion rebuilds the world for the youth.
It makes all things alive and significant."

~ *Ralph Waldo Emerson*

Ralph Waldo Emerson an American essayist, lecturer and poet. He is known for leading the Transcendentalist movement of the mid-19th century. Emerson wrote on a number of subjects including individuality, freedom, the potential of humankind, and the relationship between the soul and the surrounding world.

Do you remember when you were 10 years old? Do you remember how much energy you had? It seemed as though we would never run out of energy. It seemed as though we could play forever. Okay, I am exaggerating. Let's just say we could play for a long time. Why is that? Well, some people would argue we had the energy because we were young, and passionate about what we were doing.

Now, let's fast forward and say you are fifty, sixty, or even seventy for that matter. You could still have similar energy levels to those you had when you were a kid. The key is to identify something you are passionate about. Hey, I can watch soccer for hours and hours because I love the sport. I can also read for hours and hours because I really enjoy reading. I'm sure there are things in your life you are extremely passionate about as well. Bottom line, find your passion and you will find your inner youth!

Passion and Focus!

"Passion is energy. Feel the power that comes from focusing on what excites you."

~ Oprah Winfrey

Oprah Winfrey was born in Mississippi. She is American media proprietor, businesswoman, talk show host, actress, producer, and philanthropist. Oprah is best known for her self-titled multi award-winning talk show. She has been ranked the richest African American of the 20th century. Oprah is also considered one of the most influential women in the world.

When you are passionate about something, you are happy to do whatever it is you endeavour to pursue. I remember when I was involved in martial arts. Man, I relished the opportunity to train and rehearse my Brazilian jiu-jitsu skills. I wanted to be there. I had both passion and focus.

When you have passion and focus, you don't need anyone to light a match under you. You are, in fact, the match, and you generate your own fire. Use your passion to generate the energy you need to do what you need to do in your life, but be sure to temper it with laser-like focus, or you will be all over the place.

Passion and action!

*"We must act out passion before
we can feel it."*

~ Jean-Paul Sartre

Jean-Paul Charles Aymard was a French existentialist philosopher, novelist, political activist, biographer, and literary critic. He was one of the key figures in literary and philosophical existentialism. He was awarded the 1964 Nobel Prize in Literature, but refused it.

When I started working in Corporate America, I was an ideas guy. I could think of things no-one could think of. I was able to connect the dots more easily than most people. Man, I thought I was it. One problem, I never ended up getting consensus on my ideas, and putting them into action was almost impossible for me. Yeah, I had some great ideas by some people's standards, but I handcuffed myself by not being able to put them into action.

Eventually I learned to build consensus, and I was off to the races. There are many instances in our lives where we are passionate about certain things, but we don't follow through. We simply do not act! If you don't have a good reason for why you are not putting your ideas into motion, then you should be doing it. Don't short change yourself; act on that passion!

Passion and objectivity!

"Dispassionate objectivity is itself a passion, for the real and for the truth."

~ Abraham Maslow

Abraham Harold Maslow was born in Brooklyn, New York. He was an American professor of psychology at Brandeis University, Brooklyn College, New School for Social Research and Columbia University. He created the hierarchy of needs theory.

Ever go to a store in a mall and see that the person working there has no facial expression whatsoever? The employee has no emotion and simply does not want to be there. He/she has no passion for their work.

The scary thing is there are people all around the world who are like that. Remember, this is your life. It is up to you to create the life you want. Maybe things are less than perfect today. Maybe you thought you would be in a better position in your life. Hey, it is up to you to light that spark. Find something you are passionate about today and begin to put it into action, because tomorrow will come soon enough!

Passion and greatness!

"Man is only great when he
acts from passion."

~ *Benjamin Disraeli*

Benjamin Disraeli was a British Prime Minister, parliamentarian, Conservative statesman and literary figure. He served in government for three decades, twice as Prime Minister of the United Kingdom. Before and during his political career, Disraeli wrote romantic novels, of which Sybil and Vivian Grey are perhaps the best-known today.

Did Ghandi know he was going to be the political and ideological leader of India during the Indian independence movement? Did Nelson Mandela know he was going to lead the anti-Apartheid movement in South Africa? Ghandi and Mandela didn't know they were going to be great. They were extremely passionate in what they believed in and never swayed from that passion. They weren't looking for greatness. Their greatness came afterwards.

Each one of us can be great in our own way. I aspire to be a great husband and parent. Others aspire to be great business leaders. We will get there if we believe and are passionate in what we do. Some people don't see greatness in anyone. I see greatness in everyone. Be passionate and bring out your greatness!

Passion and balance!

"If you have only one passion in life - foot-ball - and you pursue it to the exclusion of everything else, it becomes very dangerous. When you stop doing this activity it is as though you are dying. The death of that activity is a death in itself."

~ *Eric Cantona*

Eric Daniel Pierre Cantona is a French actor and former French international footballer. He played football for Auxerre, Martigues, Marseille, Bordeaux, Montpellier, Nîmes, Leeds United and Manchester United.

Eric Cantona was a great soccer player. He was an arrogant, pompous, and self-loving, but he was a great athlete. He was a natural leader who brought the best out of his teammates, and they won as a result. In total, he won four Premier League titles in five years, and two League and FA Cup Doubles while at Manchester United.

Following his illustrious soccer career, Cantona did not know what to do with his life. Soccer consumed him, just like work consumes most of us until we retire. He, like us, really didn't know what to do next. My point here is that when you are passionate about something in your life, that's great, but when the passion is over, be sure to transition to something else accordingly. Cantona got into acting. As food for thought, what are you going to get into?

Chapter Summary

PASSION

1. Passion and commitment will enable you to succeed.

2. Without passion and energy, you have very little to go on.

3. If passion drives you, let reason hold the reins.

4. Lead the life you are capable of living.

5. Rebuild the world for the youth. It makes all things alive and significant.

6. Feel the power from focusing on what excites you.

7. We must act out passion before we can feel it.

8. Light a spark. Dispassionate objectivity is itself a passion.

9. Men and women are great when they act with passion.

10. Passion is not the same thing as obsession.

Personal Notes on "Passion"

1. _____

   _____

   _____

   _____

2. _____

   _____

   _____

   _____

3. _____

   _____

   _____

   _____

4. _____

_____

_____

_____

_____

5. _____

_____

_____

_____

Chapter 5

COMPASSION

Introduction

Compassion is a virtue. It enables us to have the emotional ability to empathize and sympathize with others given the circumstances they are in. It demonstrates our ability to connect with others for the common good. It also provides us with the sobering truth that sometimes things don't go as expected for others, and we should be grateful to have what we have.

The one thing I love about compassion is that it unites us for the common good. Unfortunately, many times we show compassion after an event has occurred. It is something that should be shown to our fellow man or woman each and every day. You can be a success in whatever you want; just have compassion for your fellow human beings, as it will do all of us some good.

Compassion and place!

"Before I was humiliated I was like a stone that lies in deep mud, and he who is mighty came and in his compassion raised me up and exalted me very high and placed me on the top of the wall."

~ Saint Patrick

Saint Patrick was a Romano-Briton and Christian missionary, who is the most generally recognized patron saint of Ireland. Saint Patrick's Day is observed on March 17, the date of Patrick's death. In the dioceses of Ireland it is both a solemnity and a holy day of obligation.

There are times in our lives when we don't perform to our own expectations. My father was a strict, but loving man. He was always my biggest supporter, especially later on in my life. I remember a time when I had three different jobs in five years. I thought to myself, what am I doing wrong? I was working smart. I was working hard. I had a great relationship with all of my colleagues wherever I worked. Unfortunately, when you are downsized, it's about business and that is life. I took it hard the very first time, because it was the first time, but my father was there for me. His words of wisdom inspired me, and they continually do so.

I know we all try to deal with the good, bad and the ugly in our lives the best way we can. We try our best to do that. After all, it's our life to lead. However, it's also nice to get compassion from someone you respect and trust, especially if it enables you to get back on your feet.

Compassion and pain!

"But my experience is that people who have been through painful, difficult times are filled with compassion."

~ Amy Grant

Amy Lee Grant is an American singer-songwriter, musician, author, media personality and actress. She is often referred to as "The Queen of Christian Pop." Having sold over 30 million units worldwide, Grant remains the best-selling Christian music singer ever.

I couldn't agree more with Grant's quote. When we go through hard times in our lives, and we will, we tend to get a different perspective on certain things. For example, some of the cities I have worked in include: Atlanta, Chicago, Detroit, and now Calgary. Moving your family from city to city is extremely difficult. Although some people are better than others with regards to change, change is something most people find difficult. It gets easier with time, but moving was still a challenge. Let's face it, there's pain associated with it.

A couple my wife and I know very well, let's call them Konrad and Teresa, lived in the same metropolitan are in the United States for over 15 years, but now they had to move. I showed a great deal of compassion to them, because I knew how difficult it would be for them. I called them as much as I could, and realized at times the change of scenery from Detroit to Dallas was extremely painful for them, at least at first. Now they are just fine, just as I thought they would be. A little compassion goes a long way.

Compassion and technology!

*"Computers are magnificent tools for the
realization of our dreams, but no machine
can replace the human spark of spirit, compassion, love, and understanding."*

~ *Louis Gerstner*

Louis V. Gerstner was born in Mineola, New York. Gerstner was the chairman of the board and chief executive
officer of IBM from April 1993 until 2002. He is largely
credited with turning IBM's fortunes around.

My daughter can type her homework assignment, speak
to someone using our home phone, text someone with
her cell phone, and go on Facebook and chat with her
friends. She could be walking next to her best friend, and
rather than talk to her, she texts her. Hey, that's the age
we are living in. She is so much into technology that it is
an extension of who she is.

This can be great because we are learning to live in this
technologically pervasive world. At the same time, it
takes us away from human contact. No machine can
replace the compassion one gives when their friend is
down, although some people believe it does. Face to face
relationships are what really count!

Compassion and rights!

*"I am not interested in picking up crumbs
of compassion thrown from the table of
someone who considers himself my master.
I want the full menu of rights."*

~ *Bishop Desmond Tutu*

Desmond Mpilo Tutu is a South African activist and retired Anglican bishop who received worldwide fame for being an opponent of apartheid. He was the first black South African Archbishop of Cape Town, South Africa. Tutu received the Nobel Peace Prize in 1984.

Compassion can be a wonderful thing. It shows you are able to feel. It shows you care about others. It shows you are human after all.

I have worked with some leaders who were focused on the bottom line. All they wanted were profits. All they cared about was money, money and more money, and nothing else. They couldn't care less about their direct reports, and in all honesty, treated them like crap. We would have a quarterly meeting and a Christmas party, and that was that.

These guys thought by throwing a Christmas party, everything was cool; well it wasn't. You may think people are stupid, but let me tell you something, they are not. Hey, you can still be bottom-line focused. You can still care about the money. Just have a little compassion for the people who work for you. A simple thing like saying hello in the morning won't kill you. Smile once in a while. Listen to the people you work with, as you may learn a thing or two. Show compassion, you will be better off for it.

Compassion and goodness!

"It would be nice to feel that we are a better world, a world of more compassion and a world of more humanity, and to believe in the basic goodness of man."

~ *Barbara Walters*

Barbara Jill Walters is an American broadcast journalist and author. Walters hosted morning television shows (Today and The View), spent 25 years as co-host of ABC's news magazine 20/20, and was the former co-anchor of the ABC Evening News. In 1996, Barbara Walters was ranked number 34 on TV Guide's 50 Greatest TV Stars of All Time.

Over the last few years there have been many natural and un-natural disasters. The 2004 Indian Ocean earthquake and tsunami comes to mind. I went on Wikipedia and it said that between 230,000 – 310,000 possible deaths resulted from this event. The day I heard about it, I was almost paralyzed. I have a family of my own and to think about all those people who passed away brought tears to my eyes.

Relief efforts were undertaken after the fact to try to help as many people as possible. The world came together to help. It's wonderful to show compassion and make a small difference in other people's lives. The earthquake and resulting tsunami which took place in the Indian Ocean provides a perfect example of that. Show compassion to people each and every day. Don't wait until it's too late.

Compassion and helping others!

"The purpose of human life is to serve, and to show compassion and the will to help others."

~ Albert Schweitzer

Albert Schweitzer was born 1875 in the province of Alsace-Lorraine, Germany (now Haut-Rhin, France). He was a theologian, organist, philosopher, physician, and medical missionary. Schweitzer's passion was to discover a universal ethical philosophy, and make that philosophy available to all of humanity. He received the 1952 Nobel Peace Prize for his philosophy of "Reverence for Life."

When I was a graduate student, I used to tutor students for free simply because they could not afford it. I really enjoyed it. Just seeing them do well on their tests put a smile on my face. It felt great because I was making a difference in someone's life!

All over the world people are helping others and making a difference. Some people volunteer as youth coaches, in soup kitchens, or at various charities. There are many ways in which we can help our fellow human beings; why not join the band wagon? You know, a little effort on your part can make a major impact for someone else. Lend a hand!

Compassion and life!

*"Too often we underestimate the power of
a touch, a smile, a kind word, a listening
ear, an honest compliment, or the smallest
act of caring, all of which have the potential to turn a life around."*

~ *Leo Buscaglia*

Felice Leonardo "Leo" Buscaglia, also known as "Dr.
Love," was an author and motivational speaker. He was
also a professor in the Department of Special Education at the University of Southern California. Five of his
books on Love were once on the New York Times Best
Sellers List simultaneously.

When I was younger I was very focused on myself.
I wanted to do well in sports, school, and life in general. I used to love to talk, and it was always about me.
Well, one day I realized it was not just about me, it was
about others as well. So, rather than talking all the time,
I began to listen, actively listen, that is. Active listening
is not a difficult skill to master, but it does take a bit of
effort on our part.

Sometimes when our kids, friends and/or co-workers
talk, all they want you to do is listen to them. Once
again, all they want is for us to 'listen' to them. I live
with three women: my wife Laureen, and my two daughters, Isabella and Victoria. I am extremely grateful they
are in my life. Although they have taught me many

things, the one thing that resonates with me is that they taught me how to listen to them. Over time, I not only improved my active listening skills, but my ability to place myself in other people's shoes. Compassion comes in many forms, one of which is active listening. You'll be surprised what a difference you can make in someone's life by simply being a sounding board. Don't talk, just listen for a change!

Compassion and helping others!

*"Have compassion for all beings, rich and
poor alike; each has their suffering. Some
suffer too much, others too little."*

~ Buddha

Siddhartha Gautama (Buddha) was said to have been
born in the small state of Kapilavastu, which is now
Nepal. He was a spiritual teacher who traveled and
taught throughout India, and on whose teachings Buddhism was founded. He was often referred to as the
Supreme Buddha. "Buddha" means "awakened one" or
"enlightened one."

Many times we get so caught up in what we do, we forget
about what is truly important. When I was younger all
I did was focus on my work. Now, I still focus on my
work, but with a higher focus on my family. On top of
that, I have increased my participation in charity events,
coaching youth soccer, and other activities. In other
words, I try to give back in some way.

Your number one priority is to take care of yourself.
Take care of your health and welfare. Once you do that,
look outside of yourself, look at the men, women and
children around you. Share your knowledge to improve
the lives of others. Show compassion and help others!

Compassion and hard shells!

*"Compassion for the friend should conceal
itself under a hard shell."*

~ Friedrich Wilhelm Nietzsche

Let's face it, there is the *'you'* who is the true you, the inner you. There is also the *'you'* who you want other people to see, the outer you. I've always been the type of guy who has worn my heart on my sleeve, so to speak. For the most part, the inner me matches the outer me. That is, the way I truly am on the inside, is the way I like other people to see me.

Many people are not like me. That is, their inside and outside don't match. Sometimes it is important to have a hard shell. An example that comes to mind is from business. The old adage is, keep business and your personal life separate if you want to succeed. The one thing I would add is to show compassion in whatever you do. There is nothing wrong with showing empathy to others, even if you are the chief executive officer of a multi-billion dollar organization. You don't have to keep that hard shell up at all times. At the end of the day we are all humans. A little empathy goes a long way!

Compassion and embrace!

*"Our task must be to free ourselves . .
.by widening our circle of compassion to
embrace all living creatures and the whole
of nature and its beauty."*

~ *Albert Einstein*

Albert Einstein was born Württemberg, Germany. Einstein is often regarded as the father of modern physics and one of the most prolific intellects in human history. In 1921 he received the Nobel Prize in Physics for his services to theoretical physics.

For one reason or another we tend to limit ourselves. We think we can't accomplish certain tasks because we don't have confidence in ourselves. We create boundaries and confine ourselves to those boundaries. We remain within the confines of those boundaries because they provide our own little comfort zone.

Every couple of days I make sure to do something that is out of my comfort zone. I despise speaking in meetings or in front of large groups. So when I get a chance, no matter how uncomfortable it may be for me, I say something to get over that fear. That is my way of breaking my boundaries. That's my way of going outside my comfort zone. It's my way of freeing myself. Once you do this for yourself, you will be more accepting of people who want to break free themselves. As a result, you will not only embrace your own personal development, but the development of others as well!

Chapter Summary

COMPASSION

1. Compassion can elevate someone to new heights.

2. People who have been through painful, difficult times are filled with compassion.

3. No machine can replace the human spark of compassion.

4. Have the full menu of rights.

5. Believe in the basic goodness of men and women.

6. The purpose of human life is to serve.

7. Show compassion by actively listening.

8. Show compassion when helping others.

9. Remove your hard shell once in a while.

10. Become free by showing compassion to yourself!

Personal Notes on "Compassion"

1. _____

   _____

   _____

   _____

2. _____

   _____

   _____

   _____

3. _____

   _____

   _____

   _____

4. _____

_____

_____

_____

_____

5. _____

_____

_____

_____

Chapter 6

PERSEVERANCE

Introduction

If you have a goal to pursue, a course of action you want to take to get to that goal, then believe in yourself, know the purpose of why you are doing what you are doing, and continuously strive to obtain your goal in a steady fashion. That's perseverance in a nutshell.

Just like baseball, life throws us a curveball once in a while. These can sometimes be challenging to overcome. I had one that almost killed me; alcoholism. It took me a while to get it under control, but now I am happier than ever. Bottom line, each of us has our own demons we need to recognize and overcome.

Above, I have shown how I have taken a personal challenge and improved my life via sobriety, but perseverance doesn't have to be about personal tragedy. Perseverance can be about reaching your greatness! That is, defining who you are, what you stand for, what your goals and dreams are, charting a course to get there, and sticking to the plan to achieve your desired goal. Bottom line, go for what you believe in and never give up! I am going to repeat those three special words: never give up!

Give a little more!

"Some men give up their designs when they have almost reached the goal; While others, on the contrary, obtain a victory by exerting, at the last moment, more vigorous efforts than ever before."

~ Herodotus

Herodotus was an ancient Greek historian who was born in Halicarnassus, Caria, which is modern day Bodrum, Turkey. Many consider him to be the "Father of History" since he was the first historian known to collect his materials systematically, test their accuracy and arrange them in a well-constructed and rich narrative.

I remember working in Chicago for a financial institution as analytics manager and researcher. I had a great time with the organization. I met some fantastic people, some of whom are still my friends today. I thought I was giving 100% in whatever I was doing, but I really wasn't. As such, my career did not prosper to greater heights. Why was that? Well, I did not want to do the selling that was required as part of the job.

I was a numbers guy. I thought those numbers would speak for themselves, but they didn't. I had to "sell" the story behind the numbers. In other words, I limited myself by not doing that little bit extra. Whether you are talking about your job, parenthood, politics, or whatever, if you truly don't give that little extra, you may not get to where you should be. Do and give just a little more; you will be surprised what you can obtain.

Never give up!

"Never give up. Never, never give up!
We shall go on to the end."

~ Winston Churchill

Sir Winston Leonard Spencer-Churchill was a British politician and statesman. He is known for his leadership of the United Kingdom during the Second World War. He is widely regarded as one of the greatest wartime leaders of the century and served as Prime Minister twice. He was an avid writer and received the Nobel Prize in Literature.

Never give up is a lesson I learned from my father, Umberto Aliberti, very early on in life. I was never the fastest or biggest soccer player, but I had 'heart' and a 'will' that would never be broken. Yeah, I would have my ups and downs, but my heart and will were never in question. I managed to earn a soccer scholarship to Oakland University and later played semi-professional soccer in Canada.

Each of us has ups and downs. Each of us gets a taste of humble pie once a while, which is fine. Why is it fine? It's fine because it brings us back to reality. If you consider it a lesson learned, it will ultimately ground you. The key is to get up from your disappointment and continue to follow your goals and dreams. Hey, there are going to be many people in your life who may challenge what you say and do, but it is up to you to never give up!

Don't get discouraged!

"Edison failed 10, 000 times before he made the electric light. Do not be discouraged if you fail a few times."

~ Napoleon Hill

Napoleon Hill was born in Wise County, Virginia. He is considered to be the most influential man in the area of personal success technique development. For more than 25 years he dedicated his life to define the reasons people fail to achieve true financial success and happiness in their lives. His book *Think and Grow Rich* has helped millions realize their dreams.

When I was younger I would make mistakes, but I would never learn from those mistakes. As I got older and wiser, I took the lessons from my failures and applied them accordingly, to the best of my abilities.

By applying what you have learned from your failures, you will ultimately reach success. If you think you don't make mistakes, well my friend, everyone does. Don't get discouraged. The next time you try to reach your desired goal, it will make it much easier to obtain. It will also make your achievement that much more satisfying.

Chart a course!

"Stay the course, light a star,
Change the world where'er you are."

~ Richard Le Gallienne

Richard Le Gallienne was born in Liverpool, England. He was an English author and poet. He started work in an accountant's office, but abandoned this job to become a professional writer. Richard is best known for writing the book *My Ladies' Sonnets.*

Do you really know what you want to do with your life? Have you defined a path or two you want to follow? Is there a passion you have that you haven't explored yet? How do you do that? Chart a course!

Start by visualizing a goal or dream that you want to come to fruition in 1, 3, or 5 years from now. Now, what you have developed is an end in your mind. Where do you go from there? First, start with the various steps you need to take and execute on to obtain your goal or dream. Next, set specific milestones you want to reach by a certain time. Last, keep your goal and dream in your mind's eye. By doing so, you will continuously reinforce where you need to go and by when. Soon enough, you will get to where you want to be. If you haven't done it already, chart your course today!

After you fall, get back up!

"Perseverance is failing 19 times and succeeding the 20th."

~ Julie Andrews

Dame Julia Elizabeth Andrews is an Academy Award winning actress, singer, and author. Andrews rose to prominence starring in musicals such as My Fair Lady and Camelot, and in musical films such as Mary Poppins and The Sound of Music. She is also an author of children's books, and in 2008 published an autobiography, *Home: A Memoir of My Early Years.*

Thomas Edison was said to have failed over 10,000 times before he developed the light bulb. Many leaders of multi-national organizations have failed miserably at various points in their careers. Parents have made mistakes providing guidance to their children. Children have made mistakes by not taking the advice of their parents. The list goes on, and on, and on.

We all make mistakes, and we will continue to make mistakes. Chalk it up to experience. The key is to bounce back. When you are down and out, get back up and continue your journey through life. If you think you are going to go through life without encountering problems, boy are you mistaken. Life rewards people who persevere, persevere, persevere, and never give up! Get it! Got it! Good!

Stay longer!

*"It's not that I'm so smart, it's just that
I stay with problems longer."*

~Albert Einstein

Albert Einstein was born Württemberg, Germany. Einstein is often regarded as the father of modern physics and one of the most prolific intellects in human history. In 1921 he received the Nobel Prize in Physics for his services to theoretical physics.

If there was any scientist I would have loved to have met, it would have been Einstein. I find his work fascinating. It takes an extremely intelligent man or woman to realize that even though they know a great deal, there is much more they do not know. Einstein himself said, "It's not that I'm so smart, it's just that I stay with problems longer."

To reach new heights in your personal development, or in life for that matter, you need to go the extra mile. Einstein realized this. I realize this. I think you realize this as well. It may not be fun and games all of the time, but the realization of your goal or dream will be worth the wait. Take those extra steps in stride; after all, they will bring you to your own personal deliverance!

This too shall pass!

"Don't let the fear of the time it will take to accomplish something stand in the way of your doing it. The time will pass anyway; we might just as well put that passing time to the best possible use."

~ *Earl Nightingale*

Earl Nightingale was an American motivational speaker and personal development guru. He was the voice in the early 1950s of Sky King, and was a WGN radio show host from 1950 to 1956. Nightingale was the author of *The Strangest Secret*, which economist Terry Savage has called "…One of the great motivational books of all time."

I have gone through some really tough times in my life, and I am sure they pale in comparison to some of the troubles others have had to endure. When we go through these difficult times, it seems as though we fall into a hole and we just keep falling, and there seems to be no way out.

When you are going through a difficult time, simply acknowledge it, accept it, develop a plan regarding how you are going to get through it, and try to enjoy the ride. After all, this too will pass!

Do the little things!

"Don't be afraid to give your best to what seemingly are small jobs. Every time you conquer one it makes you that much stronger. If you do the little jobs well, the big ones will tend to take care of themselves."

~Dale Carnegie

Dale Breckenridge Carnegie was an American writer, lecturer, and the developer of famous courses in self-improvement, salesmanship, corporate training, public speaking, and interpersonal skills. His best-selling book *How to Win Friends and Influence People* (1936) remains popular today.

I remember when public speaking terrified me. After a while I said to myself, "That's it, I'm going to take one of those Dale Carnegie course on presentation skills." It helped me then, and I have to admit, I am much better for it today. However, I still need to do the little things. Once a week I go to Toastmasters to practice and hone my presentation skills. I constantly rehearse in front of a mirror. I rehearse and modify how I can add value to each and every presentation I make. In other words, I try to do the little things that will make my whole presentation more impactful.

Life is the same way. You have to do all of the little things to get to where you need to be. Initially, those little things may be tiring and cumbersome to do, but in the long-run, you will be better and stronger for it. Let's face it, if you do the little things well, the big ones will tend to take care of themselves. What's keeping you from doing the little things?

Play until you get it right!

*"Champions keep playing
until they get it right."*

~ Billie Jean King

Billie Jean King is a former professional tennis player from the United States. King has been an advocate against sexism in sports and society. She won "The Battle of the Sexes" in 1973, in which she defeated Bobby Riggs, a former Wimbledon men's singles champion, for $100,000, winner take all. King is the founder of the Women's Tennis Association and the Women's Sports Foundation.

We can learn a great deal from Billie Jean King. Everyone thought when she had that tennis match against Bobby Riggs, she would be blown out of the water. Well, everyone who thought that was wrong.

Like Billie Jean King, in our lives we have obstacles to transcend or goals to obtain. To do this, we need to persevere and never lose sight of what is important to us. On top of that, we need to do the right things to get to where we need to be. Many times the reason we don't succeed in the things we set out to do is because we keep on doing the same thing over and over again. When you do the same thing over and over, you get the same result. Change your perspective and your attitude, and continue to persevere until you get it right. Billie Jean King did it; why don't you?

Chapter Summary

PERSEVERANCE

1. Exert a little extra effort to reach your milestone or goal.

2. Don't succumb to the distractions of life! Never give up!

3. Do not be discouraged if you fail. Everyone does.

4. Set attainable milestones and goals for yourself.

5. Perseverance is failing 19 times and succeeding on the 20th time.

6. Stick with solving life's problems. It's easy to give up.

7. Don't let fear stop you in your tracks!

8. Doing many little things is like doing one big thing.

9. Champions keep playing until they get it right.

Personal Notes on "Perseverance"

1. _____

   _____

   _____

   _____

2. _____

   _____

   _____

   _____

3. _____

   _____

   _____

   _____

4. _____

   _____

   _____

   _____

   _____

5. _____

   _____

   _____

   _____

Chapter 7

LEADERSHIP

Introduction

I have had the pleasure of working for and with some good and bad leaders. It takes time and experience to become a good leader, which is why I believe leaders are made, not born. There is a ton of literature out there about what truly makes a great leader, and the literature is pretty good. The first 6 attributes (attitude, courage, action, passion, compassion and perseverance) I wrote about in this book are some of the key qualities that distinguish a good leader from a bad one.

However, I would like to put something to rest right now that I have always wanted to say; leaders are human and they make mistakes. I don't care if you are talking about a chief executive officer of a multinational organization, a parent who is trying to do whatever he/she can to raise a family, or someone who wants to lead themselves to their full potential. All of them make mistakes.

The beautiful thing about us is that we evolve. We learn from our mistakes. What I want you to do when reading the leadership section of the book is to take the 6 attributes mentioned above and intertwine them with the different faces of leadership that I present. If you do that, you will get a better gauge of yourself from a leadership standpoint.

The last thing I would like to point out is that we all have the potential to become good, if not great, leaders. Put in the time and effort to become the leader you are destined to be!

Be a leader and visionary!

*"I skate to where the puck is going to be,
not where it has been."*

~ *Wayne Gretzky*

Wayne Gretzky is considered by many to be the greatest hockey player to ever live. He is still the National Hockey League's all-time leader in goals, assists and total points. So, what made Wayne so special? The truth of the matter is Wayne was a visionary on the ice. It seemed as though he was always one or two steps ahead of his competition.

The way Wayne executes while on the ice is the same way we try to execute each our activities each and every day. The way Wayne lived in the present during his hockey games is the way we need to live in the present at all times. Now, while Wayne was executing in the present, he always envisioned where he needed to be to make the next great play. In the same sense, while we are executing in the present, we need to envision where we need to be one, three, five years from now. This way, we take care of what needs to be taken care of in the present i.e., family, career, education, etc., while planning and executing our vision for the future.

The best leaders in every field; athletics, business, consulting, engineering, politics, and religion always focus on what needs to be done today, while developing their visions for the future. Are you one of those leaders? Are you one of those visionaries?

Inspire through Leadership!

"If your actions inspire others to dream more, learn more, do more and become more, you are a leader."

~ John Quincy Adams

John Quincy Adams was the sixth president of the United States of America. Mr. Adams stated: "patience and perseverance have a magical effect before which difficulties disappear and obstacles vanish." I am certain there were many times during his tenure when he had to be patient and persevere to accomplish his goals.

I was a soccer goalie for 30 years. To be an effective and efficient goalie you need to be both strategic and tactical, while being able to assess what is in front of you, and translate that into action for the better of the team. In other words, you have to be a leader.

There were times when we were playing against teams that were much better than us. Most people thought we would never beat these teams. You know what? We did. How did we beat these teams? The answer is actually simple; as a leader I had to lead by example. I had to believe not only in my abilities, but in the abilities of my teammates. It was up to me to motivate the team to reach the heights I knew they were capable of on game day.

Regardless of the position you hold in life, it's is up to you to believe in yourself. It's up to you dream more, learn and do more. It is up to you to bring out and become the great leader you were born to be.

Walk beside them!

"To lead people, walk beside them ...
As for the best leaders, the people do not notice
their existence. The next best, the people honour
and praise. The next, the people fear; and the
next, the people hate ... When the best leader's
work is done the people say, we did it ourselves!"

~ Lao-Tsu

Lao-Tsu was a mystic philosopher of ancient China, best known as the author of the Tao Te Ching. His association with the Tao Te Ching has led him to be traditionally considered the founder of Taoism.

To put Lao-Tsu's quote into perspective, let's imagine you are a parent. Now, let's also assume it is your responsibility to feed, clothe, instil the proper values and beliefs, discipline, educate, and ensure your siblings follow the right path towards adulthood. No matter how well you think you are doing as a parent, your children will always end up with bumps and bruises along the way. After all, that is part of life.

To lead your children, or anyone else for that matter, you need to walk beside them. In other words, teach and guide them, and let them apply your teachings and guidance. Doing things for them, or micro-managing them won't serve them well in the long-run. Use your leadership to let them grow and realize they can accomplish anything on their own.

Where do you stand!

"The ultimate measure of man is not where he stands in moments of comfort and convenience, but where he stands at times of challenge and controversy."

~ Dr. Martin Luther King Jr.

Dr. Martin Luther King Jr. was an American clergyman, activist, and prominent leader in African-American Civil Rights Movement. Dr. King was a true leader! He literally had a vision, and he motivated and moved tens of millions of Americans and people from around the world to be part of that vision along with him.

Nothing came easily for Dr. King. He had to battle racism, the status quo, as well as the social/political movement against the African-Americans in the United States. No matter where he went he was always confronted with a major obstacle. What did he do when he was confronted with an obstacle? He intelligently and strategically confronted and superseded each one.

It's easy for all of us to continue doing what we have always done. It's easy for us to get caught up in our little station in life. All of us can take a page from Dr. King's book and stand up for what we believe. We need to meet the demands of the challenges we are confronted with on a daily basis. After all, it is the true measure of who we are!

Grow yourself,
and develop others!

"Before you are a leader, success is all about growing yourself. When you become a leader, success is all about growing others."

- Jack Welch

Jack Welch was born in Salem, Massachusetts on November 19, 1935 to John, a Boston & Maine Railroad conductor, and Grace, a homemaker. He is an engineer, business executive and author. He was Chairman and CEO of General Electric between 1981 and 2001.

Jack, like all great leaders, knew he wasn't perfect. Over time, he developed his communication skills, strategic and tactical thinking, and executive presence. Personal growth was of great concern to him because it enabled him to truly refine his strengths, while simultaneously acknowledge and improve his weaknesses. Once his personal development reached a certain tipping point, he began developing other leaders at General Electric's Crotonville Management Development Centre. After all, that's what a great leader does.

Anyone placed in, or considering taking on a leadership position, has to constantly evolve to keep up with the times. Only by improving yourself can you better grow others. Jack did this at General Electric. Do you do this in your daily life?

Leadership and self-restraint!

*"The best executive is the one who has
sense enough to pick good men to do what
he wants done, and self-restraint to keep
from meddling with them while they do it."*

~ Theodore Roosevelt

Theodore "Teddy" Roosevelt was the 26th President
of the United States. He is known for his energetic personality, range of interests and accomplishments, and
his leadership. Roosevelt's achievements as a naturalist,
explorer, hunter, author, and soldier are as much a part
of his acclaim as any political position he held in office.

As one of the greatest Presidents of the United States, I'm
sure he learned a thing or two about using self-restraint
in politics. He definitely had a vision for his country, but
he had to rely on the people who worked for him to help
him realize that vision.

Whether you are the president of the United States, a
manager at a small organization, or a parent, the one
thing you want to avoid is micro-managing. By micro-
managing you are not instilling trust or empowering
people. Providing guidance so you can realize your vision
is one thing for a leader, micro-managing is another.
After all, don't you do your best work when nobody is
looking over your shoulder?

Do you elicit greatness from people?

"The task of leadership is not to put greatness into people, but to elicit it, for the greatness is there already."

~ *John Buchan*

John Buchan was a Scottish novelist, historian and Unionist politician. He is known for writing propaganda for the British war effort in the First World War, as well as being a Government General of Canada.

I'm sure that over his political career he spoke to many world leaders, which makes his quote even more powerful, as it is based on his experience. Let's take a few seconds to take his quote in, "The task of leadership is not to put greatness into people, but to elicit it, for the greatness is there already." It is here where I make the distinction between "management" and "leadership." Management is getting work done through others. Leadership is taking people where they haven't been, but need to go. That is, getting them to new heights.

If you look at leaders from every walk of life, are they really leaders? I would, without hesitation, say they are not! The majority of leaders are truly highly glorified managers. A true leader knows exactly what is in front of them. A true leader understands who they are leading.

A true leader has a vision of what needs to get done to take a vision and make it a reality. A true leader elicits greatness from those he/she leads. Once again, are the majority of today's leaders truly leaders, or are they higher level managers? Better yet, which one are you?

Don't tell them you lead!

"Being a leader is like being a lady; if you have to go around telling people you are one, you aren't."

~ *Margaret Thatcher*

Margaret Thatcher is a former Prime Minister of the United Kingdom. She was and is an extremely powerful woman. Thatcher survived an assassination attempt in 1984; her powerful stance against trade unions and her opposition to the former Soviet Union earned her the nickname of the "Iron Lady." She had clear beliefs and was articulate, confident, courageous, decisive and very intelligent. She blazed the trail for other women around the world!

Angela Merkel, the current Chancellor of Germany, is a modern day version of Margaret Thatcher. She has no need to say how great a leader she is. She has no need to show off. She knows who she is and goes about her day as one of the most powerful leaders of the world. She gets things done!

Many leaders around the globe have an insatiable urge to be in front of the camera to show how great they are. They always need to be in the minds of those they lead. They are obsessed with letting people know who they are. Most of these leaders consider themselves above the people they lead. A great leader doesn't say, "I'm a great leader," they demonstrate it through their actions. After all, actions speak louder than words.

Lead through influence!

"The key to successful leadership today is influence, not authority."

~ Kenneth Blanchard

Kenneth Blanchard is an American author and management expert. He co-authored the book The One Minute Manager with Spencer Johnson, which has sold over 13 million copies. He has co-authored over 30 other best-selling books, including Gung Ho! Turn On the People in Any Organization, and Leading at a Higher Level: Blanchard on Leadership and Creating High Performing Organizations.

First, I would like to define the words "influence" and "authority." Influence is the act or power of producing an effect WITHOUT apparent exertion of force or direct exercise of command. Authority is the act or power of producing an effect WITH the apparent exertion of force or direct exercise of command. In the past, authority trumped influence. Today, influence trumps authority.

I worked for two executives while I lived in Chicago. One always wanted to turn the world upside down. He was uptight, always felt as though he was battling for something, and gave orders. Nobody really wanted to follow him. He relied on his power to get things done. The other was calm, cool, collected and soft spoken. He knew how to sell himself, his vision and, as a result, engaged all of us. We wanted to work harder for him. He relied on influence to get things done.

It doesn't matter what career or position you are in, there are always going to be situations in which you are going to have opportunities to lead. Are you going to lead by influence or authority? Remember, the choice is ultimately yours.

Leadership and sharing credit!

"No man will make a great leader who wants to do it all himself or get all the credit for doing it."

~ *Andrew Carnegie*

Andrew Carnegie was a Scottish-American industrialist who led the expansion of the United States' steel industry in the late 19th century. He was also considered to be one of the leading philanthropists of his era.

As stated previously, in my career, I have had the pleasure of working with both good and bad leaders. I have learned equally from both types. The bad ones never really cared about the people they led. It was all about them. The very good leaders were about the people. It was about us!

I remember working for a man awhile ago. This man was extremely smart, but he always kept everything to himself. He was pompous, arrogant, and never spoke to anyone. The only time you saw him was in a meeting. By the way, most meetings were about him. He didn't realize that no matter how smart he was, he needed to get buy-in from his superiors. He thought getting a degree from a certain school automatically made you a great leader. No one truly respected his vision, no matter how smart he was. I learned more about what not to do from him, than anyone else in my life.

Great leaders are not born, they are made. They are visionaries. They illuminate their path so others can join them. They do not make people look like second class citizens. They remember to hold their needs in check, and place the needs of others at the same level, or even above their own. They make sure to bring everyone along for the ride.

Chapter Summary

LEADERSHIP

1. Always be one step ahead.

2. Inspire people through your actions.

3. As a leader, walk beside everyone, not ahead of them.

4. The ultimate measure of someone is where they stand in times of challenge.

5. Growing others will make you a better leader.

6. Leaders don't meddle.

7. Elicit the greatness that already exists in people.

8. Leaders lead! Nobody has to be told you are the boss.

9. The key to successful leadership today is influence.

10. Leaders don't do everything themselves. Share the wealth.

Personal Notes on "Leadership"

1. _____

_____

_____

_____

2. _____

_____

_____

_____

3. _____

_____

_____

_____

4. _____

   _____

   _____

   _____

   _____

5. _____

   _____

   _____

   _____

Chapter 8

HAPPINESS

Introduction

Happiness can be categorized through positive emotions. These emotions can range from being generally content to being extremely ecstatic about someone or something. Others, notably philosophers and great thinkers, believe happiness is about living the "good life."

The problem I have with all of the literature I have read is that people profess happiness is something we need to obtain. I even catch myself doing it. My next job will make me happier. If I had more money I would be happier. Once I own a better house I am going to be truly happy. Hey, it is up to us to make ourselves happy. Put things into perspective and be happy in the present! You owe yourself that much!

Grow happiness under your feet!

"The foolish man seeks happiness in the distance; the wise grows it under his feet."

~James Oppenheim

James Oppenheim was an American poet, novelist, and editor. He was the founder and editor of The Seven Arts, an important early 20th-century literary magazine. Oppenheim depicted labor troubles with *Fabian*, suffragist themes in his novel, *The Nine-Tenths* and in his most famous poem *Bread and Roses*.

Oppenheim's quote is something I can relate to directly. I used to think by getting my Bachelors and Masters degrees I would be happier with my life, but I wasn't. I used to think if I ended up getting my doctoral degree, I would for sure be happy then. Well, I wasn't. I used to think the next great job or career change would make me happy. Well, they didn't. I thought what I planned and obtained in the future would make me happy. I, without question, was absolutely wrong!

As Oppenheim states, "a foolish man seeks happiness at a distance, the wise grows it under his feet." Over the years I have learned that looking to the future for happiness doesn't get you anywhere. Now I have chosen to be wise. I choose to grow my happiness under my feet in the present; how about you?

Quality of your thoughts

*"The happiness of your life depends upon
the quality of your thoughts: therefore,
guard accordingly, and take care that you
entertain no notions unsuitable to virtue
and reasonable nature."*

~ *Marcus Aurelius*

Marcus Aurelius Antoninus was a Roman Emperor who was born in Rome, Italy. He came from an aristocratic family long established in Spain. He was also an author and philosopher. Marcus Aurelius wrote the twelve books on "Meditations."

As an emperor, Marcus Aurelius knew he would be confronted with various challenges on a daily basis. He had to be in razor-sharp form at all times. Other than a few days here and there, he knew nothing was going to be easy. After all, he was always in the public eye.

Marcus Aurelius knew the power of the quality of his thoughts. We, too, need to ensure the quality is there. If we think negative thoughts, we will behave negatively. If we think positive thoughts, we will behave positively. Our thoughts have a tremendous impact on who we are and how we live. By changing our thoughts, we will be better equipped to reach new heights. Give yourself the opportunity to reach your true potential.

Don't count your troubles!

"Man is fond of counting his troubles, but he does not count his joys. If he counted them up as he ought to, he would see that every lot has enough happiness provided for it."

~ Fyodor Dostoevsky

Fyodor Mikhaylovich Dostoyevsky was a Russian writer of novels, short stories and essays. He is best known for his novels *Crime and Punishment, The Idiot, and The Brothers Karamazov.* Dostoyevsky's works explored human psychology in the socio-political and spiritual climate of 19th-century Russian society.

Although Russia has had its problems, so has every other nation in this world. For that matter, people from every walk of life have and continue to have problems on a daily basis. Sometimes they are small problems, sometimes they are larger ones.

We can choose to complain endlessly about our troubles, or count the joys in our lives. Most people I know tend to dwell on the past, and the problems they had to deal with in the past. If you are doing so for closure, that can be a good thing. It can be detrimental if you do not give yourself the opportunity to make yourself happy. That is, if it takes from your ability to live a happy life today. Is that the case with you?

Tie happiness to a goal!

"If you want to live a happy life, tie it to a goal, not people or things."

~ Albert Einstein

Albert Einstein was a German-born theoretical physicist who developed the theory of general relativity. He is considered by many to be the father of modern physics as well as one of the most prolific intellects in human history. In 1921, Einstein received the 1921 Nobel Prize in Physics.

One of Einstein's goals was to develop the theory of relativity, and he achieved it. Einstein loved the research he did; it made him happy. The one thing we can learn from Einstein in order to reach our desired goals is to participate in things that truly make us happy.

Throughout life we make some good and bad choices. Some of those choices make us happy, others do not. Simply focus on your passion. Focus on your greatest talents. Tie that passion and your talents to a goal. Why do I say that? It's easier to reach your goal!

Keep busy!

*"The only way to avoid being miserable
is not to have enough leisure to wonder
whether you are happy or not."*

~ *George Bernard Shaw*

George Bernard Shaw was an Irish playwright and a co-founder of the London School of Economics in the United Kingdom. His major claim to fame was his innate ability to write incredible dramas. He wrote over 60 during his lifetime.

I've always wondered if Shaw came up with his quote based on his life experiences, or if he stumbled upon it while writing one of his plays. Regardless, I think we can all relate. Having time to think about things can be a blessing. The flip side of the coin is that when we do too much thinking, we become obsessed about things we have no control over.

There is nothing wrong with living in the present while planning for your future. The key is to keep yourself busy enough to enjoy the present, but not so busy as to lose sight of the future. At the same time, don't focus so much on the future that you neglect the present. Seems simple enough, but it's difficult to do.

Practice compassion!

"If you want others to be happy, practice compassion. If you want to be happy, practice compassion."

~ *Dalai Lama*

The 14th Dalai Lama is thought of as a spiritual leader. He grew up in Tibet's thousand-year-old Potala Palace in Lhasa. He lived in exile in India since the Chinese Army crushed an uprising in his homeland in 1959. In 1989, he was awarded the Nobel Peace Prize for his work advocating nonviolent means to free Tibet, his homeland, from China.

The Dalai Lama preaches compassion through his quote. Compassion is a virtue of the highest order. Through compassion we are able to get closer to our own enlightenment.

More often than not, people tend to have compassion for other people when they are going through difficult circumstances. Why wait until then? Why not show it during each and every interaction we have with others? Why not show it during the good times, too?

Happiness is linked to your values!

"Happiness is that state of consciousness which proceeds from the achievement of one's values."

~ Ayn Rand

Ayn Rand was a Russian-American novelist, philosopher and playwright. She is known for her two best-selling novels *The Fountainhead* and *Atlas Shrugged* and for developing a philosophical system called Objectivism, in which human beings have direct contact with reality through their sense of perception.

Ayn Rand was well ahead of her time, as are most true philosophers. She said, "Happiness is that state of consciousness which proceeds from the achievement of one's values." She makes the link between 'state of consciousness,' 'happiness and 'values.' That is to say, the way you perceive your world will make you happy, if what you do is tied to your values. Talk about simplicity.

I realize each of us sees the world through different lenses, but all we have to do is slightly modify those lenses so they are aligned to our values. Don't you think your happiness is worth it?

Make happiness wherever you go!

"Some cause happiness wherever they go;
others whenever they go."

~ Oscar Wilde

Oscar Fingal O'Flahertie Wills Wilde was an Irish writer and poet. He became one of London's most popular playwrights in the early 1890s. Today he is remembered for his plays and the circumstances of his imprisonment, followed by his early death.

You know, Oscar's quote is so true. Some people like to see people smile. Others live to take that smile away. Some are somewhere in between. My brother in-law, Frank, is someone who likes to make people smile. He is someone who brings the best out of me whenever I speak to him. I'm sure you have bumped into people like that.

Then there are people who are miserable. They live in a self-imposed prison. By the way, whenever they bump into you, they want you to live in it as well. The fact of the matter is that Oscar is correct; "Some cause happiness wherever they go; others whenever they go." Where do you fall?

Cheer somebody else up!

"The best way to cheer yourself up is to try to cheer somebody else up."

~Mark Twain

Samuel Langhorne Clemens, better known as Mark Twain, was an American author. He is most noted for his novels, *The Adventures of Tom Sawyer*, and its sequel, *Adventures of Huckleberry Finn*, the latter often called "The Great American Novel."

Twain knew the power of cheering someone else on. However, in today's world, we tend to do things for ourselves to get ahead. We work to obtain a goal to improve ourselves i.e., getting a university degree, a better job, or personal enlightenment. This is quite admirable. It's something special to us.

One thing I found out over time is although achieving personal goals is important to personal development, what is just as satisfying is enabling others to realize their potential. That is why I began to write. My goal is to empower people with my words. What do you do?

Choose to be happy!

"Each morning when I open my eyes I say to myself: I, not events, have the power to make me happy or unhappy today. I can choose which it shall be. Yesterday is dead, tomorrow hasn't arrived yet. I have just one day, today, and I'm going to be happy in it."

~ Groucho Marx

Julius Henry "Groucho" Marx was an American comedian and film star famed for his wit. He made 13 feature films with his siblings, the Marx Brothers. I remember watching him as a child; his quirks such as an exaggerated stooped posture, glasses, cigars, and his moustache and eyebrows made me laugh so hard.

Groucho's quote is extremely powerful. The essence of his quote is that we have the power to choose to be happy. I, like you, have met some people who, for the most part, walk around with a frown on their faces. Once in a while you get a smile out of them. I, like you, have also met people who, for the most part, are quite happy with their lives. Once in a while, you get a frown out of them.

Bottom line, it is up to you to create your day. When you wake up in the morning, you have the power and choice to be happy or not. Why not simply make the choice to be happy?

Chapter Summary

HAPPINESS

1. Be happy right now, not later.

2. Choose your thoughts carefully.

3. Count your joys.

4. If you want to live a happy life, tie it to a goal.

5. You won't know if you are happy or not if you are constantly busy. Keep yourself busy!

6. Compassion will enable you and others to be happy.

7. Happiness and values work side by side.

8. Create happiness whenever you go.

9. Cheer someone else to cheer yourself.

10. You have a choice. Make the choice to be happy.

Personal Notes on "Happiness"

1. _____

_____

_____

_____

2. _____

_____

_____

_____

3. _____

_____

_____

_____

4. _____

   _____

   _____

   _____

   _____

5. _____

   _____

   _____

   _____

Chapter 9

WISDOM

Introduction

By applying good judgment based on our knowledge and experience, we gain wisdom. Whenever I think of the word "wisdom," the following people come to mind: Buddha, Confucius, Plato, Socrates, Einstein, and Elizabeth I. Mind you, this list is far from exhaustive, and I am sure each of you could add a few names to the ones I have mentioned.

The one thing about wisdom is it is rarely something acquired at an early age. You can read many books, but the true teacher is life, the experiences it holds, and the knowledge we gain over time. More often than not, it comes from the choices we make, and applying the lessons learned from those experiences going forward.

This chapter holds some of the key things I have learned throughout my life. I placed this chapter right before the conclusion because it considers all of the previous chapters in their totality. For every page you read in this chapter, relate the information to all of the attributes I have mentioned throughout this book, and put your own spin on it. That way, you can really understand more about yourself, why you are where you are, and what you need to do to reach your potential. You'll be surprised to discover what you will figure out for yourself when you spend a few solid minutes thinking deeply about things that really matter to you. So, start reading!

Teach people to treat you right!

"Maxim for life: You get treated in life the way you teach people to treat you."

~ Dr. Wayne Dyer

Wayne Walter Dyer is an American self-help advocate, author, and lecturer. Dr. Dyer received his Doctorate in Education from Wayne State University in Detroit, Michigan. He was a professor at St. John's University prior to becoming a self-help guru.

Ever wonder why some people put themselves on a pedestal, and others think so lowly of themselves? Ever wonder why some people are more successful than others when both had the same resources available to them? Sometimes life isn't fair and things happen because they happen. It is what it is. Other times, it is about you. It is about the way you view yourself, and the way you come across. Let's face it, "you get treated in life the way you teach people to treat you." If you do not respect yourself, most people won't respect you either. It is the nature of the beast.

Take small steps each day and begin treating yourself right. Start off by defining who you truly are, based on your current value and belief system. Next, portray yourself the way you want to portray yourself to the world. This will give you the opportunity to be true to yourself, while showing the world the real you. Treat yourself with respect, and the world will be your oyster. Give yourself that gift.

Knowing is not enough;
we must apply!

"Knowing is not enough; we must apply!"

~ *Johann Wolfgang von Goethe*

Johann Wolfgang von Goethe was a German writer, pictorial artist, biologist, theoretical physicist, and polymath. His works span the fields of poetry, drama, prose, philosophy, and science. Some say Goethe is one of the most brilliant men who ever lived.

We can all learn a great deal from Goethe's quote. I am sure you have run across people in your life who have had, or still have a special talent of some sort. Some of them squander their talent because they simply do not care, which is fine. After all, that is their choice. Others simply don't want to put in the effort because they feel what they have to offer is inconsequential in the grand scheme of things.

Albert Einstein developed the theory of relativity. Can you imagine if he did not apply and share that theory with the rest of the world because he thought it was inconsequential? Making yourself small doesn't serve you, or the world, well. Why not give yourself a chance? Why not apply your talents? Let your talents shine!

Don't look for approval from others!

"Don't look to the approval of others for your mental stability."

~ Karl Lagerfeld

Karl Lagerfeld is a German fashion designer, artist and photographer based in Paris, France. He is known for being the head designer and creative director of fashion house Chanel. He owns his own label fashion house as well as the Italian house Fendi.

What a quote! If you look back at all the times you were seeking approval from others in your life, what happened? Was that pat on your back really worth it? Hey, don't get me wrong, it's great to be acknowledged. It's great to have done something special and had someone recognized your achievements. At the end of the day, though, it's what YOU think that matters.

Many of us go through life looking for approval from parents, teachers and bosses. Sometimes they validate what you have done, and sometimes they don't. When they don't it hits a sour spot for all of us, but the reality is we should have the confidence in ourselves and in our abilities to go through life on our own two feet. Don't look for approval from others; just enjoy life and approve of yourself!

Follow your bliss!

"Follow your bliss."

~ Joseph Campbell

Joseph John Campbell was an American mythologist, writer and lecturer. He is best known for his work in comparative mythology and comparative religion. His philosophy is often summarized by his phrase: "Follow your bliss."

I have worked in different cities, industries and in small, medium and large organizations throughout North America. It took a long time for me to find my true bliss. The truth of the matter is it was under my nose. I love to help people. I get satisfaction by helping people realize their dreams. Now that I have found my true bliss, I am more satisfied, fulfilled and happy.

Each one of us goes through life trying to find out what we are really good at. Some of us realize this at an early age, some of us a later on in life, and others never find out. Find out what your true gifts are. Discover where your passion lies. Follow your passion through until it becomes your true bliss! Make it happen!

Life gives tests and teaches us lessons!

"The difference between school and life? In school, you're taught a lesson and then given a test. In life, you're given a test that teaches you a lesson."

~ Tom Bodett

Thomas Edward "Tom" Bodett was born in Sturgis, Michigan. He is an American author, voice actor, and radio host. In 1997, Bodett hosted the public television program, *Travels on America's Historic Trails*. He is the current spokesman for the hotel chain Motel 6.

I worked as an automotive assembly worker for a while, and then I pursued my bachelors, masters and doctorate degrees. University taught me a lesson and then gave me a test, but working on the assembly line gave me a test that taught me a lesson.

Don't get me wrong. I have the highest degree of respect for academics. It made me who I am today, to a certain degree. However, life tests you in ways you can only imagine. The key is to take the lessons learned from your experiences and grow each and every day. My question is, do you grow each and every day from your lessons learned, or do you keep on making the same mistakes?

Paint your life your way!

"To me, the whole process of being a brush stroke in someone else's painting is a little difficult."

~Madonna

Madonna is a phenomenal singer, entertainer, and mother. Madonna has attitude, flair, is creative, and exhibits passion in whatever she does, but that is not what makes her special. What makes her special is that she creates her own world. As her quote says, "To me, the whole process of being a brush stroke in someone else's painting is a little difficult." In other words, she takes life into her own hands. Has she made mistakes along the way? Of course she has! However, those mistakes have never stopped her from reaching her desired goals and dreams.

I believe we can all take a page from Madonna's book, so to speak. Each and every one of us should wake up every morning and be a painter. What do I mean by that? Well, imagine you are a painter holding a brush, and in front of you there is a white canvas which you can paint on. Let's say the canvas represents your day. What I would like for you to do is to paint your day. This is your opportunity to create your life your way!

Whether you paint your day, week, month or years, it is you who is painting. It is you creating your life. Always ask yourself, do I want to be a brush stroke in someone else's life, or do I want to paint my life my way?

Think BIG!

*"As long as you're going to be
thinking anyway, think big."*

~ *Donald Trump*

Donald Trump, Sr. is a successful business magnate, television personality and author. He is the currently the chairman and president of The Trump Organization.

People call Donald Trump many names, some of which include: intelligent, pompous, arrogant, wise investor, real estate genius, etc.! I always see the best in people, and I call Mr. Donald Trump wise and astute. You see, Mr. Trump is the epitome of "Thinking Big." Just read his quote above: "As long as you're going to be thinking anyway, think big."

Now, although Mr. Trump coined this quote, and is definitely one who thinks big, he is not the only one who thinks big. Each and every one of us has the ability to think big. The problem is, when we get caught up in the smaller things in life, we don't give ourselves the time to think big.

How long does it take for you to think about what you really want out of life? To define your true passion? To define what truly makes you happy? In the grand scheme of things, not very long. We simply do not give ourselves the opportunity to do so.

I, for the longest time, wanted to share what I know based on my experience for the last 10 years, but I wasn't thinking big and never started a blog. Now I am writing a blog as the first step toward realizing my life's dream. Thinking small will serve you in your day to day activities. Thinking big will help you realize your life's potential!

Do something wonderful with your life!

"Being the richest man in the cemetery doesn't matter to me ... Going to bed at night saying we've done something wonderful... that's what matters to me."

~ *Steve Jobs*

Steve Jobs was the founder of Apple. The man was a true entrepreneur and visionary. Over the years, as the CEO of Apple, he amassed a tremendous fortune. In 2011, his estimated net worth was over $8 billion dollars.

On the business side, Steve was a phenomenon! He brought the Apple brand to new heights and riches. On the health side, he inspired millions of people with his mental fortitude, determination and his resounding ability to overcome tough times. Based on his experiences, Steve Jobs would definitely be a man who could provide some valuable insights to all of us regarding the true value of money.

What Steve said was that all the money in the world won't make you happy, but doing something wonderful will. Each and every one of us has a special talent, but some people have to work a little harder than others to bring it out. Why not put to work what you have to offer to the world, and create something wonderful in and for your life?

We are what we think!

"We are what we think."

~ Napolean Hill

Napolean Hill was an American author who was one of the earliest producers of personal success literature. I think he hit the nail on the head when he coined what I term the most powerful phrase in the English language. Yes, I believe "we are what we think" is a very powerful message.

I remember taking a class in Latin American studies at Oakland University in Rochester, Michigan. I was to participate in a group presentation. After the second presenter in our group finished his section, I went to the bathroom. I thought nothing of it. Then it dawned on me; this was my opportunity to leave, and I did. The rest of the group carried on, and I went to the dorm room. I let the group down, and I let myself down. This was a major defining moment in my life.

From that day onward I said to myself I would never let that happen again. I have presented in meetings where I was sweating profusely, but I continued. No matter the situation, I never gave up. Now I attend Toastmasters once a week to brush up on my public speaking skills.

We can accomplish what we want to accomplish if we are in the right frame of mind. Let's face it, if you think you can't reach your goals and dreams, more than likely you won't. If you think you will reach your goals and dreams, you likely will. Place yourself in the right frame of mind, as it will serve you better in life. After all, we are what we think!

Get comfortable being uncomfortable!

"Be willing to be uncomfortable. Be comfortable being uncomfortable. It may get tough, but it's a small price to pay for living a dream."

~ Peter McWilliams

Peter was a writer and self-publisher of best-selling self-help books. He was also a strong advocate and campaigner for the legalized use of cannabis for medical purposes.

I was an extremely shy kid growing up. I rarely raised my hand to answer any of the questions the teacher asked the class. I remember one incident in grade 5 where the teacher asked the class a question and I just hoped she wouldn't pick me. In my mind, I got so worked up over it that I started to sweat profusely. Finally the teacher chose someone other than me, and I was absolutely relieved.

Throughout my life, I have encountered moments similar to the one I just described. To be the best possible you, it is important to consider what Peter McWilliams said in the above mentioned quote. Be willing to be uncomfortable. Place yourself in situations where you are literally uncomfortable. Once you are in an uncomfortable situation, it will probably be challenging for you to remain in that situation, even for a short time. Over time, though, and with a little effort on your part, you will gradually become more comfortable.

It always starts with the first step, which is always a stretch, especially if you are trying to reach a goal you have never attained. Take that first step; it may enable you to realize your life-long dream.

Change is up to you!

*"If you don't like how things are, change it!
You're not a tree."*

~ Jim Rohn

Emanuel James "Jim" Rohn was born in Yakima, Washington in the United States. For more than 40 years he helped people shape their life strategies. Through his books and audio and video programs, he sculpted a generation of personal development trainers and top executives throughout the United States.

I remember working on the assembly line at Chrysler Canada when I was younger. Initially, I thought it was really cool. I made great money and felt as though I was living large. After a while, I realized what I was doing wasn't necessarily for me. I just wanted more out of my life. I said to myself, everything will work out in time. Unfortunately, I didn't have a plan.

I eventually I made a one-year plan. At the time, my plan revolved around completing my education. I created weekly milestones to track my progress until the day I finally graduated with my degree. Don't get me wrong, I missed a few milestones, but I never let that deter me from reaching my ultimate goal of achieving my degrees.

Essentially, I put Jim Rohn's quote into action. Hey, if you want to change, it's going to be up to you. Take that first step. You'll even surprise yourself with the things you will accomplish!

Patience and perseverance!

"Patience and perseverance have a magical effect before which difficulties disappear and obstacles vanish."

~ *John Quincy Adams*

John Quincy Adams was the sixth president of the United States of America. Mr. Adams stated: "patience and perseverance have a magical effect before which difficulties disappear and obstacles vanish." I am certain there were many times during his tenure when he had to be patient and persevere to accomplish his goals.

Now, think of the times in your life when you said you wished you were somewhere else. Think of times when you said to yourself you were not satisfied with your current situation. Think of times when you simply were not content with your station in life. Each and every one of us has encountered and will encounter those times.

The reason I like John Quincy Adams' quote so much is because it has so much practical value in life. By being patient and persevering, you will realize the fruits of your labour soon enough. The key is to align what you are doing to your values, and with your goals moving forward.

Know where you are going!

*"If you don't know where you are going,
you might wind up someplace else."*

~ *Yogi Berra*

Lawrence Peter "Yogi" Berra is a former American Major League Baseball catcher, outfielder, and manager. As a player, coach, or manager, Berra appeared in 21 World Series. He was elected to the Baseball Hall of Fame in 1972.

Each and every one of us experiences highs and lows throughout our lives. One thing I do is use a quote to stay grounded, or as present as possible, whether I am experiencing one of life's highs or lows. As such, I have started this blog on how various quotes have impacted people in their own lives. One of my favourite quotes is: "If you don't know where you are going, you might wind up someplace else." Yogi Berra, a famous player from the Major League Baseball team coined this phrase.

Every day I wake up in the morning and look at a blank wall in my home. I view that blank wall as my masterpiece for the day. What I do is use Yogi Berra's quote to create a picture in my mind, and visualize it on the blank wall. I see what I want to accomplish in my day from start to finish. I take that same approach to plan my weekly, monthly and yearly activities, goals and dreams in the same fashion. After all, if I don't know where I am going, I will definitely end up somewhere else.

If you have a quote that has impacted and improved your life in a certain way, feel free to share it.

It's what you see that matters!

"It's not what you look at that matters,
it's what you see."

~ *Henry David Throreau*

Henry David Thoreau was an American author, poet, philosopher and leading transcendentalist. The philosophical side of his personality definitely comes through his quote: "It's not what you look at that matters, it's what you see."

How many circumstances in our lives have we been in, or have been placed in, where we looked at a given situation and said, why is this happening to me? I simply cannot believe I'm in this mess? When is my life going to get better? Did you ever notice you are much more resilient than you had initially thought you would be, and your situation improved with time? Years after your experience, you may have even laughed about it.

We get upset over the smallest problems that have no true bearing on our lives or who we are as individuals. When we lose our job, it's as if we lost who we are. We diminish our value so other people won't think poorly of us. We are not as true to ourselves as we should be. We think we are never going to accomplish anything good in our lives. So what do you think we are doing? We are simply viewing everything in our lives through tainted glasses!

Look at today as the first day in your new life. Look at life through clear lenses. Wipe your glasses clean once in awhile so you can see what life has to offer, and what you are able to offer to life!

Live in and for the moment!

"To end the misery that has afflicted the human condition for thousands of years, you have to start with yourself and take responsibility for your inner state at any given moment. That means now."

~ *Eckhart Tolle*

Eckhart Tolle is the author of the *The Power of Now* and *A New Earth*. In 2011, he was listed by the Watkins Review as the most spiritually influential person in the world.

One of my favourite comedians of all time is Jim Carrey. The man has everything. He's definitely funny, wealthy, and takes life by the horns. The one thing people don't realize is that he was constantly depressed.

I say he 'was' constantly depressed because then he realized what Eckhart Tolle termed 'the power of now.' He realized he needed to live in the present, for the moment, which he currently does. Now, I'm sure Jim gets depressed once in a while, but not to the same extent as before. After all, he is human.

We can learn a great deal from Jim and from Eckhart Tolle by focusing on the present. Let's face it, the past is the past. The past is already gone, so there is no need to focus on it. We simply take the lessons learned from the past and try to incorporate them in the present moment. The future will be here soon enough. Having dreams, goals and desires for yourself is fine, but many people tend to focus more on the future than simply living life in the present.

Do yourself a favour; enjoy life now! Live in and for the moment!

Leave a trail!

"Do not go where the path may lead, go instead where there is no path and leave a trail."

~ Ralph Waldo Emerson

Ralph Waldo Emerson an American essayist, lecturer and poet. He is known for leading the Transcendentalist movement of the mid-19th century. Emerson wrote on a number of subjects including individuality, freedom, the potential of humankind, and the relationship between the soul and the surrounding world.

Ralph Waldo Emerson was an extremely wise man. I am sure he ended up gaining his wisdom from the many mistakes he made throughout his life, like most of us.

Now, most people do not like to change their direction. Many will tend to take the path of least resistance. They will take the path that has been well traveled, so they know exactly where they will be after they go down that path. Is there anything wrong with that? NO! If it is what you prefer, by all means, go that route. After all, it's convenient, easier, proven, and you are in your comfort zone.

You can take the path that is well traveled, that is, what you continually do day in and day out, achieving the same result, or take a different path and achieve your TRUE potential. Ultimately, the choice is yours! I normally take the path less traveled. What do you normally do?

Do not postpone happiness!

*"Happiness is not something you postpone
for the future; it is something you design
for the present."*

~ Jim Rohn

It seems as though most of us are rushing through life.
We rush when we are eating breakfast. We rush when we
go to work. We rush taking our kids to sporting events.
We essentially rush through life without taking into con-
sideration what we are missing in the present. Through
all of this rushing we never seem happy, even if we reach
a desired goal. Actually, we may be satisfied for a while,
but then we reach for the next goal, in a never-ending
manner.

Jim Rohn states, "Happiness is not something you postpone for the future; it is something you design for the
present." Let's use me as an example; I thought once I
worked in anything other than the automotive industry I
would be happy. Well, that was not true. I then thought,
when I get my Ph.D. in Geography, I will be happy. Well,
that wasn't true either. You see, I continued to strive for
the next goal, for the next thing I wanted in my life. I
am sure many of you can relate in one way, shape, or
form, based on your experiences. The vital component I
was missing was that I wasn't living in the present. I may
have thought I was, but I really wasn't. I realized unless
you live in the present and are fundamentally content

with who and what you are, it is difficult to be truly happy.

Hey, there is nothing wrong with creating a plan and going for your dream; just do yourself a favour and live for today. My question is, do you live in the present, or in the future?

Peace comes from within!

"Each one has to find his peace from within. And peace to be real must be unaffected by outside circumstances."

~ Mohandas K. Gandhi

Mohandas Gandhi was the pre-eminent political and ideological leader of India during the Indian independence movement. He truly believed you could solve anything through non-violence, and India was his proof.

Do you remember when you were playing with your friends when you were a kid, and you would become upset when someone took one of your toys, or did something you did not want them to do? Well, the same thing happens when you become a teenager and an adult, but the toys and circumstances are slightly different.

It's easy to get upset when something doesn't go your way. It's easy to be upset when life throws you a curveball. It's easy to just throw your hands up in the air and shout, especially when confronted with a difficult situation. However, one of the true measures of a man or woman is the ability to find peace within, regardless of the circumstance they are in. Mind you, it is easier said than done.

Exercise, meditation and reading work for me. This is how I find inner piece each and every day. It is through inner peace that I channel my energy accordingly to accomplish my daily tasks. Now, I am not saying that what I do will work for you. Each of us is unique, so you need to find out what works best for you. The distractions or circumstances of the outside world will always be there, so it's up to us to decide how we wish to respond to those distractions or circumstances.

Darkness, light and greatness!

"God gives us darkness for one reason, so that we may find the light to greatness."

~Victoria Loren Aliberti

Victoria Loren Aliberti is a grade 8 student who just wants to be a kid. Like anyone else, she has goals and dreams. It's incredible what the words of a young child yield. This quote is by far my favourite, and is the most impactful of them all.

Victoria's quote helps me put things in perspective. Hey, let's face it, life is not easy. I would be lying to you if I said it was. We bring the baggage from the past into the present. We focus too much on the future. We create our present condition. Do you see a pattern here? It's up to us to make sure we live our lives to the best of our abilities, given our current environment.

If you think about it, this quote is a culmination of all of the other quotes combined. If you believe in yourself, persevere, think like a leader and not a follower, and make wise choices, it will be much easier to get through those darker moments. Eventually, you will see the light. You will see the light to goodness. You will see the light to happiness. You will see the light that will enable you to achieve your greatness!

Chapter Summary

WISDOM

1. In life, you get treated the way you teach others to treat you.

2. Knowing is not enough; we must apply!

3. Don't look to the approval of others for your mental stability.

4. Follow your bliss! You'll enjoy your life more!

5. The difference between school and life? In school, you're taught a lesson and then given a test. In life, you're given a test that teaches you a lesson.

6. Wake up every morning and paint your day your way!

7. As long as you're going to be thinking anyway, think big.

8. It's about doing something wonderful with your life!

9. We are what we think! Nothing else needs to be said.

10. Be comfortable being uncomfortable. It's a small price to pay for living a dream.

11. If you don't like a situation, change it! You're not a tree.

12. Patience and perseverance make difficulties disappear and obstacles vanish.

13. If you don't know where you are going, you might wind up someplace else.

14. It's not what you look at that matters, it's what you see!

15. Take command and responsibility for your inner state. Start living now!

16. Do not go where the path may lead, go somewhere else and leave your mark.

17. Design happiness for the present.

18. Peace comes from within and should not be affected by outside circumstances.

19. God gives us darkness for one reason, so that we may find the light to greatness.

Personal Notes on "Wisdom"

1. _____

   _____

   _____

   _____

2. _____

   _____

   _____

   _____

3. _____

   _____

   _____

   _____

4. _____

_____

_____

_____

_____

5. _____

_____

_____

_____

Chapter 10

CONCLUSION

This may be the end of this book, but it's a time for a new beginning for all of us. We all have the power within to do some wonderful things with our lives. Why not give ourselves the power to reach our greatness?

How many times have you fallen short of your expectations? The key here is, "your expectations," not someone else's. The answer is quite simple; we all have fallen short at one time or another in our life. Now, if we have fallen short because of something that was literally out of control, well, that is life and it happens to all of us. Essentially, we learn from our experiences and move on. However, if we have fallen short for things that are within our control, well, you know who you should be looking to, to improve the outcome the next time around. Yep, it's up to you.

Your potential or greatness is something you define for yourself. Work within yourself to become a better you today. It is something that will enable you to become the person you are destined to be. I have touched on the different faces of attitude, courage, action, passion, compassion, perseverance, leadership, happiness and wisdom. As mentioned previously in this book, this list is far from exhaustive, but these attributes make a huge impact in the way we live our lives.

I feel as though I have been selfish in writing this book. Why, you say? I get satisfaction out of helping people. That satisfaction makes me extremely happy. Writing this book has enabled me to do that. It provides me with fuel to further define, refine and reach my true greatness. I truly hope I have inspired you to take your first step to the next chapter of your wonderful life. That first step to what I will term "your true greatness!"

APPENDIX

S. M. A. R. T. Action Plan

To get you on your way to achieving your greatness, I would like for you to develop a S.M.A.R.T. action plan. The letters in the acronym represent the following words: specific, measurable, achievable, realistic, and time-bound. I want you to use the key attributes mentioned in this book to develop S.M.A.R.T. goals for yourself. Following is a description of each letter in the acronym, the type of question(s) you should consider asking yourself, as well as an example for each letter of the acronym.

S = Specific: *You need to develop a very specific goal. A specific goal answers questions such as:*

- What: What do I want to accomplish?

- Why: Specific reasons, purpose or benefits of accomplishing the goal.

- Who: Who is involved?

- Where: Identify a location.

- Which: Identify requirements and constraints.

Example: I want to write an inspirational/motivational book to enable others to reach their greatness. The key to writing and publishing this work will be my daily perspective on the key attributes that I mentioned in this book, as they will enable me to do my best work to reach my desired goal.

M = Measurable: *You need to create measurable criteria that will track your progress towards your desired goal. A measurable goal answers questions such as:*

- How much?

- How many?

- How will I know when it is accomplished?

Example: I want to complete a chapter of my book every two months.

A = Attainable: *Stresses a goal that is realistic and attainable. An attainable goal answers the following question:*

- How can the goal be accomplished?

Example: I will accomplish this goal by writing 1 draft page of the book every 2 days.

R = Relevant: *A relevant goal must represent a goal that you are willing and able to work towards, and that can be accomplished. A relevant goal answers the following question:*

- Does this seem worthwhile?

Example: It is worthwhile because it will enable me to impart my knowledge on the various attributes that have had an impact on my life as well as, the lives of others I know.

T = Time Bound: *You need to establish a target date for your goal. A Time-bound goal answers the question:*

- When am I going to accomplish this goal by?

Example: I am going to complete my book on "Achieve Your Greatness" by January 2012.

So, what does my first step to <u>"Achieving My Greatness"</u> by writing a book through the use of the S.M.A.R.T. Action Plan read as? Well, following is exactly what it reads like.

S = I want to write an inspirational/motivational book to enable others to reach their greatness. The key to writing and publishing this work will be my daily perspective on the <u>key attributes that I mentioned in this book</u>, as they will enable me to do my best work to reach my desired goal.

M = I want to complete a chapter of my book every two months.

A = I will accomplish this goal by writing 1 draft page of the book every 2 days.

R = It is worthwhile because it will enable me to impart my knowledge on the various attributes that have had an impact on my life as well as, the lives of others I know.

T = I am going to complete my book on "Achieve Your Greatness" by January 2012.

INDEX

About the author

Dr. Aliberti's passion lies in helping people reach new heights, their greatness. Assisting people to realize their goals and dreams brings him true happiness.

He has a Ph.D. from the University of Western Ontario., and has previously published a book and numerous articles on mergers, acquisitions and foreign direct investment.

He currently resides in Calgary, Alberta, Canada with his lovely wife, Laureen, and his two wonderful daughters, Victoria and Isabella.

Follow him on twitter:
twitter.com/#!/VinceAliberti

Read his blog:
www.achieveyourgreatness.wordpress.com

Connect via Linkedin:
www.linkedin.com/in/vincealiberti

Send him an e-mail at:
valibert2000@yahoo.com

CPSIA information can be obtained at www.ICGtesting.com
Printed in the USA
BVOW05s0936030314

346503BV00008B/116/P